Tracy

SOMEONE FOR EVERYONE

First published in the United Kingdom in 2022 by

Canelo
Unit 9, 5th Floor
Cargo Works, 1–2 Hatfields
London, SE1 9PG
United Kingdom

Print ISBN 978 1 80032 337 7
Ebook ISBN 978 1 80032 336 0

Cover design by Emma Graves

Cover images © Shutterstock

Look for more great books at www.canelo.co

Printed and bound in Great Britain by Clays Ltd, Elcograf S.p.A.

1

For my gorgeous, funny, amazing nieces and nephews,

Love you all x

Someone for Everyone

Tracy Corbett started writing in her late twenties. As well as writing novels, she's written several short stories, pantomime sketches and magazine articles. Tracy describes her writing style as modern tales of romance, with engaging quirky characters, who overcome adversity, grow as people and conclude in satisfying optimistic endings. When she's not writing, she enjoys amateur dramatics, gardening and music. She works part-time for a local charity.

Also by Tracy Corbett

A Winter's Wish

Swept Away By You

Someone Like You
Someone to Love
Someone for Everyone

Chapter One

Kate Lawrence stared up at the Royal Courts of Justice building, with its cascade of white marble steps and Gothic Revival architecture, and felt her stomach dip. If the aim of those who'd constructed such a formidable and imposing building was to intimidate the unfortunate souls finding themselves in breach of British law, then they should be congratulated. They'd done a sterling job. She was officially intimidated.

As a solicitor, she was used to attending court. She'd represented many a client during her five-year career as a wills and probate specialist, so the idea of appearing in front of a judge shouldn't daunt her. But the cases she normally dealt with were handled by local civil courts, not by the highest court in the land.

More significantly, she'd never been the one on trial.

Her cousin Beth squeezed her hand. 'Are you sure you don't want me to come in with you? It's not too late to add me as counsel.'

Beth was also a solicitor and specialised in family law. Although she was hugely successful and earned shedloads of money, she wasn't any more suited to taking on the might of Her Majesty's Revenue and Customs than Kate was.

'I'm fine, really. I can handle this.' Kate wasn't sure who she was trying to convince more. Either way, her mouth was devoid of moisture and the shake in her legs was getting worse. 'I'm sure the judge will be sympathetic to my situation. It's not like the debts are mine.'

Beth opened her mouth to reply, but Kate cut her off before she could point out the obvious. 'I know, I'm jointly and severally liable. Legally, I'm responsible, but morally I have every right to feel aggrieved.'

'You do. And if I ever get my hands on that cheating ex-husband of yours, he'll be left in no doubt as to my feelings about the situation.'

Kate could believe it: no one messed with Beth – in court, or out of it.

Beth was a good few inches taller than Kate, her height accentuated by her elegant court shoes and immaculate grey suit. With her hair twisted up and her thick-rimmed glasses, she was the no-nonsense killer-queen of the courtroom.

If Beth was the epitome of how a successful businesswoman should look, then Kate was the slightly dishevelled version. As demonstrated when her cousin reached out and rebuttoned Kate's jacket – something she'd already done several times that morning, but the blessed thing kept popping open.

'That man's caused you nothing but heartache and pain,' Beth said, shaking her head. 'And yet he's escaped scot-free. It makes me so mad.'

'Hardly scot-free, Tristan's declared himself bankrupt.'

Beth pinned her with a look. 'Only so he could avoid paying his debts and leave you to clear up his mess. Selfish bastard. And he's hardly riddled with guilt, is he? He buggered off and impregnated another woman, after telling you for years he wasn't ready to have kids. The man's beyond reproach.'

Harsh words, but Kate couldn't argue against them.

A rumble of thunder vibrated through the chilly air, adding to the gloom.

'I'm sorry, Kate. Come here.' Beth drew her close and hugged her. 'I'm just so angry on your behalf. I want to throttle the man. I hate the way he's hurt you and jeopardised your career. It makes my blood boil.'

Despite struggling to breathe, Kate allowed herself to be consoled. 'Getting angry won't help anyone,' she mumbled, her

2

face squashed against Beth's collarbone. 'What's done is done. The divorce has been finalised, so he can't hurt me anymore. I just need to get this last debt sorted and then I can start over.'

'Assuming the judge doesn't side with HMRC.'

Kate pulled away from Beth's embrace and unearthed a tissue. 'I have no control over that, other than to plead my case and hope for leniency. At least once it's over, I'll know what I'm dealing with.'

'Let's hope you're right.' Beth's concerned expression indicated she wasn't as confident as Kate of a positive outcome. 'But if the judge doesn't show leniency, please don't panic, okay? You can stay with me as long as you need to. It's not a problem. I'm here to support you until you're back on your feet.'

'Thanks, Beth. I wouldn't have coped without you these past few months, but I don't want to outstay my welcome. You and Matt want to move in together and get a place of your own. I don't want to be the reason you can't do that.'

Beth waved away Kate's concerns. 'Nonsense! We're happy to take our time. Matt isn't going anywhere.'

As evidenced by the number of times he stayed over.

But Kate didn't mind. She was pleased for her cousin; everyone deserved that kind of love and commitment, and Beth had certainly found it with Matt Hardy. It was just sad that it hadn't worked out that way for her.

Her smile faded when she checked her watch. 'It's nearly time, I'd better go in.'

'Are you sure you don't want me to come in with you?' Beth buttoned up Kate's jacket for the umpteenth time. 'Or I could wait out here? I don't mind.'

'I'm fine, really. I have no idea how long I'm going to be and you have a client meeting at four. Seriously, go home. I'll be okay.'

Beth hugged her. 'Call me as soon as you're done.'

'I will.'

3

Beth kissed her cousin's cheek. 'Be strong. And remember to cry, especially if it's an older male judge. Try to look vulnerable and broken.'

Something that Kate didn't feel would take too much effort. She'd felt permanently broken for the last two years, ever since that night when she'd woken at three a.m. to find Tristan's note on the bedside table detailing the full extent of his debt situation. A situation she was jointly responsible for – even if she had been kept in the dark. Ignorance was no defence, not in the eyes of the law.

Waving Beth goodbye, Kate took a deep breath and climbed the multitude of steps leading up to the imposing courthouse. She felt slightly sick. Her hands were clammy and her legs barely had enough strength in them to manage the climb. By the time she reached the top, she was light-headed and even more unbalanced on her court shoes.

Maybe wearing a suit hadn't been such a good idea: a casual outfit would have been more likely to evoke the judge's sympathy. Unlike her tall and slim cousin, Kate's physique wasn't built for containment. Her bum was disproportionately big compared to the rest of her and strained against the tight skirt, creasing it in all the wrong places. But if she bought a larger size then the waist would be too baggy. Her shirt never stayed tucked in, and she was forever walking out of her court shoes.

Still, if she failed to avoid bankruptcy today, her law licence would be revoked and her career would be over, so she'd never need to wear a suit again. Every cloud, and all that.

Checking the summons letter, she headed into the grand lobby and queued to be scanned at the security machines. The case was being heard on the first floor of the Thomas More Building, room 110. She looked around at the array of medieval signs, but couldn't see the room listed.

Conscious of the time, she asked for directions and was sent through the Queen's Bench Division, across a courtyard and

4

into a side annex, where she finally arrived at her destination. Unlike the grandeur of the rest of the building, room 110 was a dump, with dull beige flooring and matt grey walls, enhanced by stark furniture that wouldn't have looked out of place in a prison.

The clerk sitting behind a desk didn't look up when she approached. 'Name?'

'Kate Lawrence.'

'Representative's name?'

'I'm representing myself.'

He glanced up and gave her an appraising look. 'Fill this in,' he said, pushing a form in front of her. 'The hearing's scheduled for two o'clock.'

'Not too long to wait then.'

'Along with eight others.'

Kate's stomach dipped. It looked like she was in for a long afternoon. 'Thank you,' she said, heading for one of the plastic chairs.

The room was eerily quiet and uncomfortably cold. Having filled in the form and returned it to the clerk, she settled down and inserted her earphones, hoping some music might help to relax her.

Closing her eyes, she dropped her head against the wall and pondered how she'd ended up here, broken-hearted, alone and facing financial ruin.

Her mum had been so proud of her when she'd won a place at university to study law. It had felt like the breakthrough they'd both needed – an escape from struggling to survive – to a life filled with promise and financial security. Her dad's suicide when she was a baby had shaped them both, bringing them closer together in one sense, yet keeping them apart in another.

Her mum had been forced to work several jobs to pay the bills, so Kate had spent most of her childhood being looked after by Aunty Connie and Uncle Kenneth in Godalming.

She'd envied her three cousins, with their loving parents and big house and regular holidays abroad. She'd craved siblings of her own and a dad who would teach her to swim and ride a bike, but instead she'd worn second-hand clothes and relied on free school meals, and her first holiday abroad hadn't been until she was well into her twenties. Her only luxury had been music lessons, paid for by her aunt and uncle.

Luckily, she'd been close to her cousins, especially Beth. Megan was an actress and Alex was… well, he was still making up his mind what he wanted to be, but hopefully he'd get there soon. Sadly, her aunt and uncle had now separated, so there were no more family gatherings to attend, but she hoped her relationship with them would remain unchanged.

Despite her own fall from grace, at least her mum had found happiness. Marrying Brian had brought her stability, security and love, and it was no more than she deserved. Now all Kate had to do was sort out her own life.

If she'd known it would be gone four p.m. before she was called into the chamber, she'd have gone to the loo. Even the dulcet tones of Lewis Capaldi on her phone hadn't distracted her from the sight of the other defendants being ushered into the room, returning a while later looking forlorn and downcast. By the time her name was called, her mouth was drier than the bottom of a budgie's birdcage.

The court clerk showed her into the chamber, his bowed head resembling the stance of a funeral officiant, which didn't bode well.

Despite the dullness of the room, the judge wore the full regalia: long sumptuous robes with a huge velvet collar and infamous starched curly wig. In contrast, the representative from HMRC wore a shabby suit and scuffed shoes. At least, she assumed he was her opposition. He looked fed up, tired and not in the mood to play 'friendly', which did nothing to calm her nerves.

The clerk gestured for her to sit down. No sooner had she done so, when the judge banged his gavel and announced the start of proceedings, causing her to scurry to her feet.

The judge checked her name and address, before turning to the HMRC representative. 'Mr Whittle, you have applied for an application of bankruptcy?'

'Yes, Your Honour.'

'I'm assuming all efforts to secure engagement with the defendant and agree on a repayment schedule have been exhausted?'

'Yes, Your Honour.'

The judge scribbled something down. Without looking up, he said, 'Can I assume by your attendance today, Ms Lawrence, that you wish to contest the application for bankruptcy?'

Kate cleared her throat. 'Yes, Your Honour.'

'On what grounds?'

'Compassion, Your Honour.'

The judge looked up from his pad. 'Compassion?'

The HMRC representative smothered a smirk, believing his case to be already won.

The judge frowned at her. 'That is not one of the directives available to me, young lady. I can adjourn an application if there is good reason. I can challenge the plaintiff's efforts to engage in reasonable negotiations to repay the debt, and I can ensure the evidence is admissible and that the proper process has been followed. What I cannot do is overturn an application for bankruptcy if all attempts to recover the debt have failed and the defendant is liable for that debt.'

'I understand that, Your Honour. But I also believe I'm allowed to petition the court to deny bankruptcy if the debt can be repaid to the creditor.'

'That option should already have been explored. Are you saying you're now in a position to repay the debt?'

'No, er... I mean, yes, but not within the timeframe HMRC are allowing. I need longer to pay off the debt, which is something I'm very keen to do. Bankruptcy would result in my licence to practise law being revoked and that's something I'm desperate to avoid.'

The judge raised an eyebrow. 'You're a solicitor?'

'Yes, Your Honour. I specialise in wills and probate.'

He looked down at his file. 'I can't see any details of your salary listed. Are you currently employed?'

'It's a bit complicated—'

'With all due respect, Your Honour.' The HMRC representative jumped up. 'We're fully aware of Ms Lawrence's personal circumstances and a thorough financial assessment has been carried out. Our conclusion is that Ms Lawrence has insufficient means to repay the debt within a reasonable timeframe.'

The judge removed his glasses. 'I have no doubt that due diligence has been carried out by your office, Mr Whittle, but I will allow the young lady a few minutes to enlighten me.'

The man didn't look happy, but didn't query the matter further and sat down.

Kate rubbed her clammy hands on her skirt, trying to control the shaking. 'Thank you, Your Honour. The debts were accrued by my ex-husband during our marriage. I was unaware of their extent – or that a number of them had been taken out in joint names – until after bailiffs had been instructed to recover the debts. Over the last two years, I've made a concerted effort to pay off the money owed and avoid any legal action, which until three months ago I believed I'd achieved.'

The judge replaced his glasses and checked his file. 'There is a property listed here – has that been sold?'

'The flat is currently being repossessed by the mortgage company and there's no equity. I'm temporarily living with my cousin in Godalming, where I'm working as a paralegal for my uncle's family law firm.'

'A paralegal?'

'Yes, I was previously employed by Blandy & Kite in Putney, as a wills and probate specialist.'

'Was your position terminated?'

'No, Your Honour, but I couldn't afford to stay in London. I felt that moving back in with family would allow me time to find another job and rebuild my life, even if it meant a demotion. However, I'd never have given up my job in London if I'd known that money was still owing to HMRC.'

The judge lifted a document from the file. 'The debt owing to HMRC covers unpaid tax and fines from self-employed earnings for five years. Are you claiming you were unaware of these debts?'

'Yes, Your Honour. My ex-husband led me to believe the business he ran was registered as a limited company. That's the only reason I agreed for my name to be included as a director.'

The judge referred to his notes again. 'I see that your ex-husband has declared himself bankrupt.' He turned to the HMRC representative. 'Have sufficient attempts been made to recover the debts from Mr...' he glanced at his notes, 'Mr Morrison?'

'Yes, Your Honour. Mr Morrison is living in a local authority property and claiming Universal Credit. His partner is also unemployed. We have no expectation of him being able to repay the debt within the foreseeable future.'

The judge turned to Kate. 'Which rather leaves you in a precarious situation, does it not, Ms Lawrence?'

'Indeed, Your Honour. However, my intention is to find another job and clear the debt as soon as possible. I just need more time.'

The judge tapped his glasses with his pen. 'I'll allow an adjournment of three months.' He checked the calendar on his desk. 'A new hearing will be scheduled for the beginning of February. If by that time I am satisfied you're in a position to repay the debt in a reasonable timeframe, say two years, then the application for bankruptcy will be suspended.'

'But Your Honour...' HMRC man didn't look happy.

'That is my final decision. Case dismissed.' He banged his gavel on the desk and offered Kate a sympathetic smile, before exiting the courtroom.

The HMRC representative packed up and left without comment.

Kate took a moment to catch her breath, before picking up her bag and following him.

She'd done it: she'd successfully persuaded the judge to allow her more time. It wasn't the perfect outcome – three months wasn't very long – but it was better than nothing. Now all she had to do was find a decently paid job in the hope she could resolve her debt situation – something she prayed would happen soon.

It was dark by the time she emerged from the courthouse. Rain pelted the grimy London streets, splashing water against her legs as she headed for the tube station. Apprehension and a nervous state of anxiety had made her hot and clammy prior to the hearing, but spent adrenaline and acute disheartenment had left her shivering and cold in the November night air.

She sped up, eager to get home and soothe her sorrows with a long hot bath and an equally large glass of something laced with gin; she was in need of an anaesthetic.

A noise behind her made her glance over her shoulder, but there was no one there, only a few shadows darting across the wet pavement. The trees in the neighbouring cemetery rustled in the breeze, as if whispering conspiratorially, but it was just her imagination playing tricks on her; no one was following her.

She turned off the main road and into a side lane, trying to shake off the tension clamping her skull and making her head ache. Her shoulders were like cement, rigid and unrelenting – a symptom of a stressful day.

She just prayed another panic attack wasn't looming. She'd managed to keep a lid on her anxiety so far today, but the constant threat of a meltdown lurked beneath the surface, poised and ready to strike.

As she made a mental note to stop off and buy painkillers, a dark figure lunged out from behind the wall and grabbed her arm, knocking her off balance.

Shock caught her off guard and her immediate instinct was to hit out. Her fist connected with the assailant's chin, making a crunching sound, which was followed by a low moan. This wasn't enough to deter the man, who was wearing a black balaclava and thick gloves – something which sent a wave of fear racing through her.

As they grappled, the man shouted at her, spitting in her face. 'Bag! Now!'

Realisation dawned. She was being mugged.

The sensible lawyerly part of her brain told her to let go of the bag. Losing a few possessions wasn't worth the risk of getting hurt, but another part of her refused to let go. Why, she wasn't sure. She clung to the straps, pulling against the man as he dragged her down the lane.

They staggered one way, and then the other, like some bizarre tug-of-war contest. Kate was losing ground; the man was clearly stronger. If she was going to fend him off then she needed to fight dirty. She kicked out, missed him and stubbed her toe on the wall behind. Sudden pain almost made her lose her grip, but the rage burning within her fuelled her strength and she wrenched the bag as hard as she could.

The bag slipped from the man's clasp, causing her to stumble backwards. She lost her footing and fell hard onto the wet pavement, banging her head against the concrete as she landed with a thump.

The next thing she knew, the man was above her, kicking her in the ribs as she cowered on the pavement. 'Give me the bag,' he barked, his black padded jacket failing to mask his body odour. 'I won't ask again.' And then he drew a knife.

Oh, hell.

Once again, Kate's sensible lawyerly brain told her to give it up as a lost cause, but she was damned if she was going to let another male lowlife take something else from her. All the pent-up anger that had been bubbling under the surface for the last two years finally exploded in a torrent of aggrieved outrage.

'Or what?' she yelled, swinging her legs around and catching him hard on the kneecap. 'You'll stab me?'

He staggered backwards, allowing Kate to scrabble to her feet.

'Quite frankly, after the year I've had you'd be doing me a favour, mate. You want my bag? You seriously want my bag?' She shook the thing at him. 'Do you know what's in it? Do you?'

He waved the knife at her. 'Just give me the bag!'

'I have precisely twelve pounds and thirty-three pence!' She ripped open the bag and pulled out her battered purse. 'As you can see... there are no credit cards, store cards or charge cards... Why, you ask? Because they've already been cut up! You are, however, welcome to take my library card and my donor card... although perhaps I should hold on to this, seeing as you're about to stab me! At least that way I can do something useful and save the life of some poor sod awaiting a liver transplant!'

The man hesitated. 'You're mad, you are.'

'Mad?' Kate let out a scream. 'I'm frickin' furious!'

'Just give me the bag!' He sounded slightly desperate now.

Kate stamped on the ground, jarring her already sore foot. 'You are not taking my bag, do you hear me?' She swung the bag and hit him with it. 'Do I make myself understood? I'm sick to death of selfish men thinking they can take whatever they want. Use me. Expect me to pay off their debts and then bugger off with another woman!' It felt good to release some of the rage that had been building since that day when bailiffs had turned up on her doorstep.

She stood there defiantly, with her hands on her hips. 'So go on then, stab me.'

The man must have sensed she wasn't backing down and he ran off, sporting a bit of a limp, which did at least give her some satisfaction.

'Nutter!' he shouted back, before disappearing round the corner.

'Right, 'cause I'm the one who's unhinged!' she yelled after him.

And then the pain registered with her brain. A tsunami of signals flooded her senses, alerting her to her battered state. Her foot hurt from kicking the wall, her chest hurt from the sudden burst of unaccustomed exercise and her ribs ached from being kicked.

With no fight left in her, she collapsed against the wall and slid to the ground, panting and clutching her ribcage. Wet seeped through her suit jacket and increased the intensity of her shivering. It was official: her life could not possibly get any worse.

Then she reached up and felt the back of her aching head, and a wave of nausea flashed through her when she saw the blood. She tried to stand, but the queasiness made her dizzy and she had to lean against the wall to steady herself.

However badly she was hurt, she had to get home. If she waited around any longer, it would only be a matter of time before some other lowlife took a pot shot at her and finished her off completely.

Staggering back up the lane, doing a first-class impression of a drunken football hooligan, she briefly wondered whether she should call the police. But what could she tell them, other than he had a London accent and body odour? It would be just another unsolved crime, a statistic to add to the many other attacks that occurred on the city's streets.

As her chest tightened and her breathing turned ragged, she dug out her phone and called her cousin.

Above her, a firework exploded into the night sky.

Remember, remember, the fifth of November.

Well, she wasn't likely to bloody-well forget it, was she?

Chapter Two

Tuesday, 16th November

When The Rose Court Care Home came into view, Calvin Johnson slowed to halt and gazed up at the grey stone building, with its tall ornate windows and eerie Gothic roofline. A sense of dread settled over him, as he anticipated what awaited him inside. If he'd known what being the executor of his great-uncle Bert's estate entailed, he would have stayed in Leeds and not agreed to take it on, but it was too late now: he was stuck with it.

His plan had been to pick up his uncle's paperwork and return to his home town within a day of arriving. But that was before he'd realised his uncle's records predated electronic storage. Instead of a few files and uploading stuff onto memory sticks, he'd discovered piles of dusty old ledgers filled with his uncle's loopy handwriting – beautiful to gaze at, but totally indecipherable. He couldn't even fit a third of the ledgers into his Mazda coupe. They filled an entire room – and not a small room: a huge period library with floor-to-ceiling bookcases that required one of those stepladders on wheels to reach the top.

He'd also found the place in a state of disrepair and with only a handful of staff looking after the residents. Watching their acute exhaustion as they tried to manage everything meant there was no way he could just turn around and leave. Which was why he was still here, regretting getting involved and desperately trying to find a solicitor prepared to take on the case, so he could escape back to Leeds.

He walked through the iron gates and past the gargoyle statues perched on matching stone pillars. They were ugly things, with pointy ears and razor-sharp teeth. Not exactly a fitting advert for a care home, even if it did fit with the area's spooky reputation.

The quaint village of Pluckley was filled with a range of period oast houses and historical buildings. The kind of place that attracted ramblers, and people with an interest in National Trust properties and afternoon teas. It also claimed to be England's most haunted village, housing seventeen resident ghosts – one of which lived in the care home – hence the gargoyles: a warning to anyone approaching.

The care home had formerly been a hunting lodge, built in the early sixteenth century, and had housed various dukes and baronets over the years. Nestled in the Kent countryside, and surrounded by woodland and fields, it was certainly an appealing place to spend your latter years. Sadly, such an old building required a lot of upkeep and expense, and as he was discovering, there was no money – only debts.

Hanna Wozniak was waiting for him the moment he stepped over the threshold. The large wooden door creaked on opening, so it was impossible to sneak in undetected – something he'd discovered during the last three days, when he'd done his best to avoid the formidable head nurse. She was like a bloodhound, determined and unrelenting.

He'd only managed to sneak out this morning because she'd been preoccupied with handing out medication to the residents and hadn't seen him sliding out the back door. It wasn't exactly brave, but he'd needed space to get his head around the gigantic problem that had landed in his lap. A problem that seemed to be growing in magnitude with every new piece of information he discovered.

'You avoid me,' Hanna said, her Polish accent the only indication that English was her second language. She was standing with her arms folded across her chest. 'We need to talk. You not leave again. I need answers.'

Except he didn't have any answers, only more questions – like how he was supposed to apply for probate when he didn't understand the forms and he couldn't find a solicitor willing to take on the case.

All the law firms he'd approached had declined to offer representation, waffling on about 'billable hours' and 'no liquid assets'. On paper the estate had a decent amount of equity, including several leasehold flats in London, a few garage blocks and the care home property in Kent, which alone was worth a packet. But that wasn't enough to persuade the solicitors, who had wanted a hefty retainer upfront – something he didn't have – to compensate for months of hard graft before seeing any commission.

'I have list of grievances,' Hanna said, producing a piece of paper from her pocket. Her jet-black hair was shaved on one side and dyed bright blue – the same blue as her nurse uniform. Her eyes were lined with black kohl and her ears had several piercings, the silver chains linking each one like chain mail. With her deathly pale skin and thick dark eyebrows, she looked scary as hell. But the residents loved her, and he'd been assured that she wasn't as fierce as she appeared, but he wasn't convinced.

'Staff not paid for five months. *Five months,*' she said, holding up five splayed fingers, like he couldn't count. 'How do you expect us to live?'

'I'm really sorry,' he said, knowing it was a feeble response, but unable to offer anything more useful. He'd done nothing but apologise since he'd arrived, but he had no idea what he was doing. Something which was becoming acutely apparent to the care home staff who, he realised, had hoped his arrival signified the end of their woes. If only. 'As soon as funds become available, everyone will get paid, I promise.'

'When? I need date.' Hanna blocked the doorway, preventing him from evading her questions.

To the left of the lobby, the dining room was laid out ready for lunch. Each table was set with proper cutlery, linen napkins

16

and vases of fresh flowers. No matter how bad things had got, the staff team hadn't let the residents suffer, and that just made him feel even guiltier. He really needed to do something – he just didn't know what.

'I honestly don't know,' he said, with a shrug. There wasn't any point in lying to her. 'I'm struggling to find a solicitor to help me with the case.'

'Not good enough. You have money, yes?' She looked him up and down, assessing his branded clothing. Hugo Boss polo shirt, Nike cargo trousers and top-end trainers. 'You footballer. You earn big salary. You pay staff.'

The sinking feeling that had haunted him since his diagnosis in June returned. Everything tightened within him – his stomach, his brain, his throat – and he had to fight back the emotion threatening to surface.

Maybe it would be easier if his body ached or flinched with pain occasionally. If his precision when striking the ball wasn't so effortless, it might soften the blow of losing his career. In twelve years of playing professional football, he'd never suffered from repeated injuries like some of his teammates. He'd trained eight hours a day, six days a week, enduring cardio sessions, strengthening exercises, shooting drills and hours of practising free kicks, and his body had never once let him down.

And then, out of the blue, the GPS vest they wore during training to monitor heart rates and recovery times had flagged up an irregularity. Further investigations had resulted in a diagnosis of hypertrophic cardiomyopathy – HCM, as it was more commonly known. A condition that thickens the walls of the heart muscle and can affect the heart's electrical system.

Whether he was born with it or it had developed with age, the doctors couldn't tell him. The only thing they could be certain about was that his career was over. Extreme exercise could cause his heart to stop at any moment and result in sudden death, and that wasn't a risk that the club or the Football Association was willing to accept. So, despite never having had any symptoms, or even a twinge in his chest, his dream was over. Just like that. And he had no idea how to deal with it.

'I'm no longer a footballer,' he said, swallowing back the pain in his throat. Even saying the words aloud hurt. 'I'm unemployed.'

And it wasn't just professionally that he'd been sidelined. Prior to his diagnosis, Ainsley had been the perfect girlfriend, loving and loyal. Post-diagnosis, she'd become 'unsatisfied with where the relationship was heading', which had been news to him. He hadn't wanted to believe that the change in her feelings was linked to his career ending, but it was hard not to draw that conclusion, especially as she was now dating one of his teammates.

Hanna gave him a disdainful look. 'You tell me you have no savings?'

He was embarrassed by the line of questioning. 'Not enough to cover the salaries of the entire staff team and ongoing expenses of running a business, no.'

He'd stopped any unnecessary spending the moment he'd been forced to retire. He'd never been stupid with money; he'd always kept within his means, but that was a moot point when faced with someone who hadn't been paid for five months and whose annual salary was less than he'd earned in a week as a footballer. She had every right to be fed up.

If he'd known that his career would be cut short, he'd have made different decisions. As it was, he'd invested most of his earnings, just like the financial adviser had told him to. He'd bought a house in Leeds, bought shares in various companies and paid heavily into a pension scheme, knowing his retirement would come earlier than in most professions. He just hadn't anticipated it being at the age of twenty-nine.

Much to the horror of the financial adviser, he'd also bought his mum a house, paid for his two younger siblings to attend university and bought them flats to help them get ahead in life. These didn't constitute 'sound financial decisions' apparently. It was 'lost money'. But maybe if the bloke had experienced the upbringing Calvin had, he might think differently. His dad had left when he was eight – disappearing back to Jamaica – forcing his mum to work several jobs to put food on the table. If it hadn't been for Granny Esme and Great-uncle Bert stepping in to help when things got really bad, life would have been a lot worse. There was no way his conscience would allow him to earn shedloads of money and not help his family out.

But just as Uncle Bert's wealth was tied up in investments and property, so was his.

'How you expect us to pay bills?' Hanna wasn't letting him off the hook.

He frowned. 'I thought you lived at the care home?'

'Me live here, yes. Natalie, too. We get fed, we not live in gutter. But you think we don't have bills? Natalie have baby, she use food bank for nappies and clothing.'

His stomach dipped. Natalie was the other nurse and she worked nights; she was also trying to support a nine-month-old baby single-handedly. 'I didn't realise Natalie was using a food bank,' he said, ashamed to be standing there in his expensive clothing when one of the nurses was reliant on handouts. He knew first-hand what it was like to rely on charity, and it wasn't a good feeling. 'I'll get her the stuff she needs for the baby.'

'What about other stuff?'

There was more? He might as well hear the worst of it. 'What else is on your list?'

Hanna read through the items. 'We have no maintenance person to fix broken things. No admin person to run place. No activity coordinator to keep residents happy. And CQC rating is poor. If no better by January, place get closed down.' She made a slicing motion across her neck. 'Dead in water. What happen to residents then?'

He didn't like to point out that the place might have to close anyway, regardless of another inspection. There were only three options available to him. Sell the business. Liquidate it. Or take over running the place – something he had absolutely no intention of doing, even though his uncle had presented it as an option in his will. Calvin was utterly bemused as to why his uncle thought he had the right skill set to run a care home. He didn't have the aptitude, abilities or experience. All he knew how to do was kick a bloody football. But he didn't feel it would be helpful to enlighten Hanna about the precariousness of the care home's future. Not yet, anyway.

Until yesterday, he'd never heard of a CQC rating. He now understood it to stand for Care Quality Commission, an assessment of the care-home standards. Standards they were failing to meet, putting the residents at risk, which was adding to his feelings of inadequacy.

'And we have no hairdresser or chiropodist,' Hanna continued, shaking the list at him. 'They not get paid, so won't come. Residents begin to look like werewolf. Long hairs and nails.' She made a claw with her hand. 'Residents also need physio. We have bedbound patient, Priya. Priya need physio to stop bedsores.'

He rubbed his forehead, desperately trying to calculate how much he had in savings. Was it enough to pay for physio visits? If not, he'd have to cash in one of his investments; he couldn't let the situation continue. 'I'll sort something out, Hanna. I promise.'

'Good. And soon. Situation not acceptable.' She took a step closer and pinned him with her heavily kohled eyes. 'And we need two more nurses.' She gave him the V sign, emphasising the need for two extra people, but there was no mistaking the intention behind her rude gesture: she was making a point. 'Two. Okay? No cover for sickness.'

And with that she marched off, leaving him feeling like he was standing on the brow of the *Titanic*, watching his life sink into the icy-cold Atlantic below.

He'd thought his life couldn't get any worse.

Turns out, he was wrong.

Chapter Three

Friday, 19ᵗʰ November

Kate stared up at the place she'd once called home, seeing it as it truly was: an uninspiring, generic high-rise flat in the heart of Clapham. The brown cladding was ugly and the sky-blue panels inserted below the glazing dated back to the 1970s, when the place was built. The weather didn't help. It was cold, grey and drizzling. A dismal day to match her mood. She could almost feel her fine blonde hair frizzing and slipping from its clasp, as if it wasn't up to the fight either.

It was a world away from how she'd felt when she'd first moved here. She'd been so excited to own her first home. A foot on the property ladder, with all the promise of good times ahead and leaving the struggles of her childhood behind. Fast-track five years down the line and she was in worse financial strife than she'd ever been in as a child. They might have struggled for money when she was younger, but her mum had never allowed them to get into debt. Now Kate was clinging on to solvency by the skin of her teeth and sinking under the weight of bills that never seemed to stop piling up. At least after today she'd never have to set foot inside the wretched place again. It was the only thing keeping her going.

Pulling her long navy cardigan around her, she headed inside the uninspiring building.

As usual, the lift stank of cigarettes and stale urine, but at least it was working today and she didn't have to climb the four flights of stairs several times to collect the last of her belongings.

Thankfully, Beth had loaned Kate her car, so she didn't have to lug everything home on the train. It was the last opportunity she had to take anything of sentimental value, before handing over the keys to the mortgage company.

The front door of her flat needed a shove to get it to open. Further dread settled over her when she saw the pile of post stacked up on the doormat, brown envelopes stamped with red slogans announcing: 'Do Not Ignore'. Tempting as it was to burn the lot, she knew that wouldn't make the problem go away.

Kicking off her wet boots by the door, she skimmed through the envelopes, relieved to note that most of them were addressed to Tristan. Their divorce had severed their financial connection, so any debts in his sole name were now his responsibility alone.

She paused when she discovered one addressed to her, an official-looking letter from Mordens Collection Agency. *What did they want now?* She'd cleared the Council Tax debt, hadn't she? She'd discovered that trying to manage escalating debts was like trying to hold on to sand. Debts would frequently be sold on, passing from one collection agency to another, each one adding their own interest charges and instructing bailiffs to call. Bailiffs who refused to take no for an answer, and would threaten to remove goods and issue a warrant for her arrest if she didn't comply. Dealing with them had been intimidating and incredibly frightening.

With a shudder, she gathered up the letters and shoved them in a bin bag. She'd deal with them later – today was depressing enough without adding to her stress levels.

Looking around the small space, she could see that Tristan had visited since the last time she was here. The TV and Sky box had gone, as had the John Lewis lamp that her mum had given them as a moving-in gift. *Nice of him to help himself.* Why was she even surprised? He'd taken everything else from her, including her self-esteem – a floor lamp paled into insignificance by comparison. All that was left was the cheap Ikea sofa and her beloved upright piano.

Sadness gripped her as she went over and lifted the lid, running her fingers over the keys. It hadn't been an expensive instrument, only fifty pounds from Gumtree. She'd love to keep it, but the storage costs would be too high and she couldn't ask Beth to house a piano.

Sliding onto the stool, she played a few chords – minor keys, of course, melancholy to match her mood. Talk about self-pity. She let out a self-deprecating laugh and began playing Chopin's funeral march. In public, she tried to put on a brave face. It was only when she was alone that she allowed herself to wallow.

She hadn't always been this way – although she'd never been an extrovert, she'd been open and honest and trusting. Optimistic, even. She took people at face value and believed them to be who they were. When she'd met Tristan at university, she'd had no idea he'd turn out to be so... reckless. He'd seemed so mature for his age, so focused and driven. He'd had big ambitions and seemed to want the same things she did: a good career, a nice home and a family one day.

Her playing grew louder, the keys vibrating under her hands as she bashed out the chords, remembering how the debts had started piling up. Tristan seemed unable to stick to a monthly budget, and became resentful and challenging when she tried talking to him about it. And then she discovered he was gambling online. The next thing she knew, debt collectors were turning up at the door, demanding immediate payment, and life as she'd known it was over.

A knock on the door startled her.

She stopped playing. Had she been too loud? Was it a neighbour complaining?

And then she realised she was crying. When had that happened?

Another knock on the door.

'Hang on, I'm coming,' she called out, guessing it was the mortgage company arriving early.

Another rap on the door.

'I'm coming!' she called out, her agitation levels increasing. As she yanked open the door, the sight that greeted her sent her stumbling backwards and she immediately slammed it shut again.

A wave of panic raced through her as she leant against the door, her heart pounding in her chest. There was no way that man was from the mortgage company. He must be a bailiff, or a debt collector. Why wouldn't they leave her alone? Hadn't they taken enough?

She jumped when there was another knock.

Turning, she squinted through the spyhole and assessed the man standing on the other side. Medium height, bronze-coloured skin, with a neatly trimmed goatee. His Afro hair was longer on top and tied up, a contrast to the fade-to-skin shaved section beneath. Sleeve tattoos covered his arms and his lean athletic physique was visible beneath his short-sleeved black top. He was definitely not a representative from the mortgage company. Not unless NatWest had significantly changed their uniforms.

'What do you want?' she called through the door. 'I don't have any money and there's nothing valuable in the flat.'

She saw him frown. 'Excuse me?'

'The mortgage company have repossessed the flat,' she said, struggling to control the shake in her voice. 'Legally, you're not allowed to take anything. It no longer belongs to me.'

'Why would I want to take anything?' He sounded genuinely bemused, but she wasn't falling for his act. She'd been here before.

'That's what people like you usually want.'

'People like me?' His frown deepened. 'What does that mean?'

The shaking in her hands increased. 'I know you're only doing your job, but you have no idea how intimidating it is to have people forcing their way into your home.' All the bad experiences she'd encountered over the past two years came flooding back and her chest started to contract.

'I'm not forcing anything.' He looked down the landing, as if searching for backup.

'Only because I haven't opened the door. The minute I do, you'll stick your foot in the gap and prevent me shutting it. I know how it works.' Beads of perspiration began to trickle down her face. She tried slowing her breathing, but she began to feel dizzy. This wasn't good.

The man rubbed his forehead. 'I'm here because I need some information about the lease on the flat.'

Kate paused. Was it a trick? 'I don't believe you.'

He lifted his hands. 'Why would I lie?'

'To get me to open the door. I've fallen for lies like that before.' But a slither of doubt crept into her psyche. He didn't look like the men who usually showed up here – he was too trendy for one thing. 'Who do you work for?'

'No one. My name's Calvin Johnson. My late uncle owned the freehold for this block of flats and I'm trying to find out who owns the individual leases.'

She tried to compute what he was saying, but the rushing in her ears made it hard to focus. No one would make up such an elaborate lie, surely?

Holding herself steady, she cracked open the door a fraction and peered out. 'Do you have any ID?'

He removed an expensive-looking leather wallet from his back pocket and produced a driving licence. She noticed a designer watch circling his wrist and an Armani logo on his top. He was definitely not from the mortgage company.

Regret began to surface. 'You're not a bailiff, are you?'

His eyebrows lifted. 'You thought I was a bailiff?'

'I'm sorry, I made an assumption.' She opened the door, stung by mortification. 'It's just...' She knew what she wanted to say, but the words got stuck in her throat and a fresh batch of tears exploded. 'Bailiffs keep... showing up... and demand letters arrive... and then the court hearing...' Her chest grew tighter as she tried to explain. 'I was attacked... and it's all got a bit much...' The room grew darker and she realised she was about to pass out.

She slumped against the door frame, struggling to breathe, unable to exhale.

Closing her eyes, she tried to stem the onslaught of a panic attack, but the throbbing in her head and the sense of nausea that washed over her overrode any attempts to quell the inevitable.

The next thing she knew, she was falling. She braced herself, but before she hit the floor with a thud, she was caught and half-carried, half-dragged over to the sofa.

'It's okay,' the man said, lowering her onto the seat. 'Try to relax. You're safe.'

A warm hand gently rubbed her back as she fought for breath.

'Slow breaths, that's it. Relax your hands.'

Her hands? Her nails were digging into her palms. Right, hands. Relax. She loosened her grip and stretched them out.

She conjured up an image of sitting in front of an open fire, her feet curled under her, reading a historical romance as the snow drifted down outside. *Focus on your happy place*, she told herself, like the mental-health nurse had instructed.

As her breathing slowed, her senses slowly sharpened... which would have been fine, had she not been sitting on the sofa of her repossessed flat with a man she didn't know, who was continuing to rub her back.

He must have sensed her tense under his touch, because his hand suddenly disappeared, leaving a cold void where it had once been.

He stood up and moved away. 'Keep breathing slowly,' he said, disappearing out the door as if he'd been an apparition.

Silence descended and she was alone again.

She should have felt relieved.

The man had turned up uninvited and spooked her. She had every reason to feel aggrieved. But did she really? He'd done nothing wrong. She'd jumped to the wrong conclusion and assumed he was from a collection agency. Why hadn't she apologised? Or explained? Instead, she'd burst out crying, hyperventilated and collapsed in a messy heap. She was officially a disaster.

A noise startled her. She glanced up to see the man reappearing through the door.

'I left the door ajar,' he said, coming over. 'I didn't want you having to get up. I got these from the shop downstairs.' He handed her a box of tissues. 'I also got you this.' He handed her a takeaway cup. 'It'll help relax your airways.'

She accepted the carton. 'You seem to know a lot about this.'

'My brother had asthma as a kid. Do you have an inhaler?'

She glanced away, embarrassed. 'It's not asthma…' she trailed off, not wanting to admit that she suffered panic attacks. There was nothing to be ashamed of, but she hated losing control, especially in front of strangers. She took a sip of the drink and the velvety taste of chocolate hit her senses. 'You got me hot chocolate?'

He gave a half-hearted shrug. 'I figured you'd need something sweet.'

Was the man a mind reader? She wasn't sure whether to be grateful or alarmed. Both, probably. Either way, she was glad of the drink. 'Thank you, it's really kind of you.' She'd forgotten his name… Kevin? Keith? Calum?

'No worries, is it helping?'

She nodded and took another mouthful. 'You can sit down, if you'd like.'

'Okay.' Except there was nowhere to sit, other than on the solitary sofa – the rest of the furniture had disappeared. He looked apprehensive about sitting close to her again, so perched on the arm of the sofa. A moment later, he said, 'Were you really attacked?'

She stared down at her lap; it was easier if she didn't look at him. 'A couple of weeks ago. I was on my way home from a court hearing and a man tried to take my bag. I managed to get away, but it shook me up.'

'I'll bet. Were you hurt?'

'Not badly. Bruised ribs, a mild concussion. But it's left me a bit... unnerved.'

'Understandably.' His voice was soft, and she noticed he had a northern accent. Yorkshire, maybe. 'You said you'd been in court?'

It seemed strange to be sharing her woes with a stranger, but he'd been so kind to her, and the least she owed him was an explanation for having misjudged him. 'I was defending an application by HMRC to make me bankrupt. I managed to persuade the judge to allow me more time, but he's only given me three months to find the money. And it's a lot of money, nearly ten grand.'

He whistled. 'Tough ask.'

Her chest began to tighten and she tried to rub away the ache. 'Luck hasn't exactly been on my side of late.' She grabbed more tissues and tried to stem the onslaught of further tears. 'They're not even my debts.'

He reached over and took the cup from her so she could blow her nose. 'You don't have to tell me, if you don't want to.'

'I need to, so you don't think I'm a horrible person.'

He drew back, alarmed. 'Why would I think that?'

'Because I jumped to conclusions when I saw you and assumed you were a bailiff.' She shifted to face him. 'It's just that my ex-husband had a gambling problem, which became worse when his business got into trouble, and then he started covering up the extent of the issue by lying and borrowing money from payday loan companies.' She sucked in a breath, trying to draw in enough air to continue. 'And then after we'd split up, bailiffs started showing up. They've taken all my jewellery and valuables; they even seized my car... and threatened to have me arrested if I didn't pay up.'

'Jesus, you must've been so scared,' he said, sounding genuinely sympathetic and looking sheepish. 'And then I show up. Sorry.'

'It's not your fault, really. I haven't been here for months. I only popped in today to pick up the last of my things and hand over the keys to the mortgage company. I thought I'd be okay, but all these bad memories came flooding back… and, coupled with being mugged, I guess I panicked when you knocked on the door. I made a horrible assumption, and I feel awful. I'm so sorry.'

He hesitated, as if his instinct was to go to her again, but he thought better of it and stayed put. 'Honestly, no harm done. It was my fault for turning up here. I did send letters, but not everyone replied, so I thought I'd visit in person.'

'Your letter's probably in that bag,' she said, nodding at the bin liner.

He offered her the takeaway cup. 'Want some more?'

'Thanks.' She took the hot chocolate, grateful for something to sooth her scratchy throat. 'You said you needed information on the flat lease?'

'That's right.' He shook his hand, loosening the fancy watch on his wrist. 'My uncle died a few months ago and I'm trying to sort out his estate.' His hands came to rest in his lap and she noticed beautifully manicured nails. And she'd thought he was bailiff? What an idiot she was. 'He was an architect back in the day and he designed a load of tower blocks in London. He retained the freehold on some of the buildings, but I can't get a value until I know who owns the leases and whether any of them have been extended.'

Kate sipped her hot chocolate. 'Wouldn't you be better off using a solicitor? Leases can be complex.'

'I can't find anyone willing to take on the case.'

She frowned. 'Why not?'

'All the money's tied up in property and I can't afford an upfront retainer. There's no available money to pay a solicitor until after everything's sold, and that could take months.'

'That is a problem,' Kate said, feeling bad for him – it was a common scenario. 'When I worked for Blandy & Kite, we were limited as to the number of cases we could take on that wouldn't generate immediate income. I'm sorry, it's not fair, I know. I can sympathise.'

For a moment he seemed baffled. 'Are you a solicitor?'

It was no wonder he seemed surprised. She hadn't exactly displayed professionalism, or even sanity. 'Yes, although right now I'm working temporarily as a paralegal, until I know whether I have a career left or not. If I'm made bankrupt, then it's game over.' She snatched at another handful of tissues, willing herself to stop crying.

He was still looking at her. 'What area of law do you specialise in?'

'Wills and probate.' She took another sip of hot chocolate and forced a smile, for her sake as much as his. 'Why, do you want to engage me?'

'Yes.'

She stilled. 'I was joking.'

'I'm not. I'm desperate, and by the sounds of it, so are you.' He repositioned himself next to her on the sofa, not touching, but close enough that she could see speckles of copper in his brown eyes. Calvin. That was his name. Calvin Johnson.

She swallowed awkwardly, unsure where this conversation was headed – and slightly thrown by his close proximity. 'You want me to apply for probate for your uncle's estate?'

'Yes, I do. I'm the executor and I have no idea what I'm doing. I really need the help. And it's a big estate, so your fee will be substantial. As well as the tower blocks in London, there's a few garage blocks and a large property in Kent. The commission will easily clear your ex-husband's debt.'

She liked that he hadn't referred to it as her debt. 'There must be a catch?'

'Several.'

She almost laughed. He was honest, she'd give him that. 'Go on then, hit me with it.'

'All the records are stored in handwritten ledgers dating back to the 1950s. I'm struggling to find out who owns the leases on the all the flats, and the property in Kent is a care home. There are several debts and the staff there haven't been paid for five months.'

That didn't sound good. 'Who runs the business accounts?'

'My uncle did.'

She was almost afraid to ask her next question. 'No one since?'

He shook his head. 'It's a bit of a mess.'

An understatement. The chances of her dealing with an estate of that complexity in three months were slim-to-none. Valuing the estate alone could take years.

But what other choice did she have? This was the first glimmer of hope she'd had in months to escape her predicament. This had the potential to solve her problems, even if not straight away. Her uncle would allow her the time off, she was sure of it. He hadn't really needed a paralegal; he was just helping her out, so she wouldn't be missed.

She held out her hand. 'You have yourself a deal.'

He let out a sigh of relief. 'You have no idea what this means to me.'

When he shook her hand, she almost sighed, too, but for an entirely different reason. His grip was so warm and soft, it was almost as comforting as the hot chocolate. Thankfully, she stopped herself in time.

'Hopefully, it helps us both out,' she managed to say, aware she'd yet to release his hand, and unsure as to why. Maybe she was distracted by his hair, which she'd noticed faded from a dark chocolate brown colour to almost blond at the ends.

'I'm Kate Lawrence, by the way,' she said, fighting for professionalism and not allowing herself to be distracted by the man sitting next to her.

Something that proved impossible when he said, 'Kate Lawrence, you're a lifesaver,' and his face broke into a huge smile. The impact nearly had her falling off the sofa, and for the second time that day she lost her breath.

It was rude to stare open-mouthed at someone, but she couldn't look away, even if she'd wanted to. His whole face changed when he smiled. His eyes creased, his dimples turned from slight dents into deep crevices that framed his even white teeth, and his face just… Well, it glowed. There was no other word for it. It was like the sun coming out on a cloudy day.

A sense of foreboding settled over her and she quickly withdrew her hand. Getting all doe-eyed over a man was not what she needed, or wanted. She was still recovering from her marriage imploding. No man was ever going to burn her like that again. Not ever.

She would not allow herself to be distracted by a man with an adorable smile and cute dimples… however nice, and genuine, and sincere he appeared to be.

Especially, when that man was now her client.

Chapter Four

There had only been a couple of times in Calvin's life when he'd felt genuinely apprehensive about something. He'd always been so assured about who he was and what was expected of him. He knew what he needed to do to achieve success and he had direction in his life, a clear path ahead. But all that had changed back in June, when he'd been given his diagnosis. Now he felt nothing but doubt and uncertainty. He questioned every decision, second-guessing himself, and felt consumed by remorse when he dwelled on the ramifications of certain choices – like hiring Kate Lawrence as his solicitor.

He'd had a knot the size of a football in his stomach all weekend, thinking about how he might have made his situation worse, and not better. But it wasn't like he'd had a choice, was it? She was his last resort. He never usually made rash decisions, and maybe he wouldn't have done it she hadn't been so endearing. But when she'd looked up at him, all wounded and fragile, through those watery blue eyes, he'd melted. He just hoped he wouldn't live to regret it.

And now he had to face another demon, this time in the shape of the care-home chef, Geraldine Henderson. Something else he wasn't looking forward to tackling.

Geraldine hadn't been in work last week; she'd been prescribed bed rest following a steroid injection in her hip, and an agency chef had been hired – the fees for which Geraldine had covered herself. He couldn't imagine this endeared him to

33

the woman, or eased the concerns of the rest of the staff team that things were about to improve any time soon.

He tapped on the kitchen door, unsure about intruding on her workspace. Chefs were notoriously territorial about their domain, as Hanna had already prewarned him. 'Don't piss off chef,' she'd barked, pointing a purple fingernail at him. 'We need food. Not survive without. Be *charming*.' A threat that hadn't helped to ease his trepidation.

He wasn't sure he knew how to charm a seventy-nine-year-old woman, but then he thought of his granny Esme and instantly felt calmer. Her train was due to arrive in an hour and he couldn't wait to see her. Hopefully, she'd help him sort out this mess and placate the staff, because he wasn't resolving anything on his own.

'Hello,' he called out, pushing open the door. 'Is it okay to come in?'

The kitchen was a big room, with exposed brickwork, a high ceiling and huge sash windows. An Aga was situated next to an open fireplace, which had a load of pots and pans hanging down from the hooks above. A thick wooden table filled the space in the centre and was covered with various baking ingredients.

Geraldine turned at the sound of his voice and he braced himself for another confrontation, but she surprised him by smiling. 'Calvin, love! Finally,' she said, limping over, her apron covered in flour. She pulled him into a tight hug and squeezed him. She smelt of pastry and lemons. 'I've been dying to meet you. Let me look at you.' She held him at arm's length and made a point of checking him over. 'You're quite the looker, aren't you? I bet you don't have any trouble getting the ladies.' She pinched his cheek. 'And I thought your great-uncle was handsome.'

This wasn't what he'd been expecting. But then, feeling dumbstruck was becoming a common occurrence. 'It's lovely to meet you, Geraldine.'

She was a good foot shorter than him, with soft curly brown hair and one of those cheerful faces that instantly put you at ease. He could relax; she was no Hanna.

He held out his hand, but instead of shaking it, she cupped his face with her floury hands and kissed him right on the lips. Another thing he hadn't been expecting.

Thankfully, it was brief, and she instantly pulled away. 'You daft thing, you're almost like family. No need for such formality.' She was still holding his face in her hands. 'Would you like a cuppa?' She wiped his cheeks, removing smudges of flour. 'Silly me, I've got you all messy.'

He took a step back, dislodging her hands before she spat on a tissue and began wiping his face like his granny used to do when he was little. He wasn't up to that level of intimacy. 'I'm good, thanks. How's your hip?'

'A bit sore, but it'll never be right until they replace it, so I just have to make the best of it.' She gave her hip a pat, still smiling, even though it must be painful being on her feet all day.

He was consumed by another wave of guilt. 'I'm really sorry you've been put in this situation, Geraldine. Hanna said you'd intended to retire by now. I hate that you're being forced to stay on to help us out.'

She gave him a stern look. 'Firstly, no one's forcing me to do anything, and secondly… wait a sec…' When a dog barked, she headed over to the back door. 'I promised Bert I wouldn't leave until you were settled and had found a replacement. I'm not reneging on my promise,' she said, opening the door and letting in a large dog.

The animal was a lanky blonde thing, who trotted over to Calvin and sat obediently in front of him, gazing up with huge brown eyes. Calvin reached out and stroked the dog's fluffy ears. 'That's incredibly kind of you, Geraldine, but that doesn't mean you're expected to use your own money to keep us afloat. Hanna tells me you buy all the food for the care home.'

Geraldine dismissed his concerns with a wave of her hand. 'What else am I going to do with it? I live alone, I have no family and the money's just sitting there gathering sod-all interest. I'd rather put it to use. Besides, in case you hadn't realised, the care home has no money. I'm not going to sit back and watch the staff and residents starve, am I?'

She had a valid point, but still. 'I promise to pay you back as soon as possible.'

'No rush, my love,' she said, filling a bowl of water in the deep ceramic sink. 'You concentrate on getting to grips with running this place, we're relying on you to get it back to how it was in your uncle's day.'

That was what worried him. He still had no idea why his uncle had chosen him to deal with the estate. He wasn't the obvious choice, by a long shot.

'Your uncle used to talk about you all the time,' Geraldine said, placing the bowl of water in front of the dog. 'He was so proud of you. He watched all your football matches on the telly, said he knew you'd make it big the first time he saw you kick a ball.'

Calvin felt a lump in his throat. 'He was a nice man.'

'He was quite the lover, too,' Geraldine said with a wink. 'This is Suki, by the way. Suki the Saluki. Do you like dogs?'

But Calvin was still reeling from the realisation that his uncle and Geraldine had been… intimate. 'Er… yes, I do.'

'She's a smashing dog. Loyal as anything, and a right soppy thing. But she needs more exercise than I can manage these days. Do you know much about Salukis?'

'I don't.' He looked down at the dog – with her pretty, slim face and long floppy ears covered in wavy fur – and was instantly reminded of Kate Lawrence. Not that she had floppy ears, but she had the same wounded, doleful expression, as though life had given her a good kicking. He couldn't imagine she'd thank him for comparing her to a dog, so he'd keep that observation to himself.

.'This one's a rescue animal, so she's a bit damaged, poor thing.' Geraldine produced a treat from her apron pocket. 'A complex mixture of nervous sensitivity and clumsy exuberance. Of course, she's also beautiful, elegant and extraordinarily agile.'

Yep, that definitely described Kate Lawrence. He'd never seen anyone faint so gracefully.

The dog sniffed at the treat and knocked it to the floor, before looking up at her owner as if fearful she was about to be told off.

'Daft thing.' Geraldine held on to the table as she bent down to retrieve the treat. 'Not as agile as Bert, mind you. He was quite the flexible gentleman.'

Which wasn't something Calvin needed to know. 'Probably too much information, Geraldine.'

She hauled herself upright, laughing. 'You're not embarrassed, are you?' She looked at him intently. 'Oh, goodness, you are. Look at those adorable cheeks, they've gone all pink. How funny. That's the trouble with you millennials – you think you invented sex. Let me tell you, it wasn't called the Swinging Sixties for nothing.'

Calvin rubbed his chin, unsure how to react to the details of his great-uncle's sex life. And to think he'd been nervous about being shouted at. 'I had no idea you and Uncle Bert were so close.'

'No reason why you should. He was a discreet man, your uncle.' She patted his cheek. 'He was also determined to ensure you and your family were looked after, which is why I owe it to him to support you all I can.'

Calvin felt his heart soften. He'd always got on well with Uncle Bert; as well as teaching Calvin how to swim and play cricket, he'd also taught him how to use a power drill and change a plug socket. Skills he'd never seen the need for, but his uncle had told him that life wouldn't always be about football and he'd need something to fall back on. Maybe his uncle had known what was coming.

'Thanks, Geraldine. I appreciate it, but I don't want to take advantage, so if the situation ever changes, let me know, okay?'

She made a cross over her chest. 'You have my word.'

Calvin checked his watch. 'I have to go and pick up Granny Esme from the station, but is there anything you need from me? Anything I can help with?'

'You can take Suki for a walk whenever you get the chance. That would definitely help me out. The poor girl's a ball of pent-up energy, she's fit to burst. And we all know how frustrated a woman gets if she doesn't get a regular fix, right?'

Calvin had no idea what the appropriate response was to that, so he opted for, 'No problem, I'll take her out later when I get back.' He gestured to the door. 'I'd better be off – it was great to meet you, Geraldine. And thanks again for your support. I'm forever indebted to you.'

'Ah, away with you. You'll make me come over all unnecessary.' She squashed him into another hug. 'Goodness, you're solid,' she said, her hands feeling down his back. 'I like that in a man.'

He held himself rigid, afraid to move. Even the dog was looking up at him with a wide-eyed expression, as if embarrassed by her owner's behaviour.

'Right, enough of that,' Geraldine said, eventually extricating herself from the hug. 'Work to do, cottage pie to make.' And with that, she limped over to the Aga and busied herself with the cooking. 'Bye, love.'

Calvin left the kitchen, wondering who would prove to be the more challenging to deal with – Hanna and her fierce demands, or Geraldine and her wandering hands. He didn't relish either.

Pluckley train station wasn't far away, but his granny was eighty-three and not as active as she once was, so he made the short drive into the village and parked up in the forecourt out front.

He was a few minutes early, so he climbed out of the car and wandered over to watch a group of kids playing football in the school playing field.

Resting against the fence, he smiled when the football soared into the air and landed in a deep puddle, splashing up muddy rainwater. The kid in him still had the urge to jump the fence and run to join in with the game.

He'd always been the same, constantly running around kicking a ball – before school, after school, every weekend. He'd lost count of the times his mum had appeared and tapped her watch, reminding him it was late and he had homework to do. He hadn't cared about schoolwork. The only thing that mattered was football.

Deciding he'd tormented himself enough, he returned to the station to wait for the train to arrive. There was no guard, so he walked onto the solitary platform to wait.

He checked his watch. In his old life, he'd be having a wellness check now: the medical team would be assessing his blood and urine, and setting him a gym programme to complete after the morning training session. Instead, he was living in rural Kent and feeling like he'd taken hallucinogenic drugs that had transported him to a parallel universe.

Part of him had been glad to leave Leeds and escape the town's enthusiasm for the beautiful game. A frenzy of fans had followed the team with a dedication that was obsessive, and he still had people come up to him in the street and ask for his autograph, expressing their sorrow for his situation and wishing him well. It was genuine, he knew that, and he was grateful for their kindness. But he also knew that the adoration would soon fade. Give it another year and he'd be forgotten, a player only a few would remember.

He had no qualifications, no other skills, no other passions. It had only ever been football. How was he supposed to move on from that?

The train appeared in the distance and slowly chugged to a halt. A couple of doors opened and few people disembarked, but not his granny. He was just wondering if she'd missed her train, when she appeared further down the platform, struggling under the weight of a heavy holdall.

He jogged to reach her, took her bag and placed it on the ground so he could hug her, but she pointed to the train. 'Can you get the others?'

Others? How many bags did she have?

He hopped onto the train to find three suitcases wedged into the cycle rack. 'Which one's yours?'

'All of them.'

He turned to her. 'All three?' How long was she intending to stay?

A whistle blew further down the platform.

His granny flapped her hands about. 'Quick, before the train pulls away.'

'They won't pull away while the door's still open.' At least, he hoped not. He lifted the suitcases onto the platform. 'Is that everything?'

'Yes, love. Thank you. Now come here and give me a hug.'

Granny Esme was almost as tall as him, with long silver hair that she wore in something called a 'chignon', which made her look like Patsy from *Absolutely Fabulous*, his mum's favourite show. A pair of bright blue wide-framed glasses perched on her nose; they were too big for her face, but she insisted she needed them for 'peripheral' vision.

'It's good to see you, Esme. I've missed you.' It still felt odd using her name, without the prefix of 'granny', but the word had been banned now that all her grandkids were adults. The word was 'ageing', apparently, and on the rare occasion it slipped out, he'd be quickly reprimanded. Publicly, he obeyed. Privately she would always be Granny Esme.

'I've missed you, too, my love. How are you?' She pinned him with her sharp brown eyes, a concerned look on her face. It was a look he was used to.

Grandad Charlie had died when he was a baby, and when Calvin's dad had returned to live in Jamaica, his granny had

40

moved in to help look after him and his two siblings while his mum went out to work. It was Granny Esme who'd taken on the school when they'd wanted to reprimand him for skipping classes to attend football training, and it was her who'd accompanied him to Armley Road to sign his first professional contract with Leeds Park United. She'd been there for all the big milestones in his life, including the time following his HCM diagnosis, when he'd cried for three whole days, so there was no point lying to her – she knew him too well.

'Not as bad as I was,' he said honestly, kissing her powdery cheek. She always wore 'rouge', as she called it, and was never seen without her rose-coloured Chanel lipstick. 'The care home's in a bit of a mess. I didn't realise how bad things were.' He balanced the holdall on top of one of the suitcases and extended the handle. 'I'll have to come back for the third suitcase. My car's parked out front.'

Esme fell into step next to him, looking smart in her bright green trench coat and matching scarf. She'd always been quite the style icon. 'I was worried that might be the case. Bert's health hadn't been good for years, and I suspected he wasn't keeping on top of things. Have you managed to find a solicitor to help you?'

He kept his eyes focused forwards. 'I have.'

'Well, that's something. A local firm?'

He swallowed awkwardly. 'No… an independent, a woman called Kate Lawrence.' He walked through the station and onto the forecourt, speeding up slightly in the hope of diverting the conversation elsewhere. 'There's my car over there.'

Esme caught him up; she was still nifty on her feet. 'An independent? Is that usual?'

Opening the small boot, he debated how much to say. Was it better to prewarn people that he might have made a monumental mistake and hired a woman who suffered from panic attacks and was in even more of a financial mess than he was? Or would it be better to stay quiet and hope for the best?

It wasn't like it was Kate's fault. She was grieving for the loss of her life – a situation he could definitely relate to. He knew what it was like to have the rug pulled out from under you. And although he had his concerns about her state of mind, it wouldn't be fair to share her woes with anyone else; it wasn't his place. She'd only told him because he'd ambushed her. Keeping quiet was the respectful thing to do, and certainly the safer option, since the staff were jittery enough as it was.

'Long story,' he said, lifting the suitcase into the boot. 'The good news is that she's between jobs, so she'll only be working for us and hopefully it won't be too long before we can apply for probate. She's arriving this Thursday.' He wheeled the second suitcase around to the driver's side, hoping it would fit in the back seat. The two-door coupe was not designed for carrying excessive luggage.

Granny Esme watched him struggle to squeeze the suitcase behind the driver's seat. 'Will she be staying at the care home?'

'It seemed like the best option. I can't pay her until after probate is complete, and a hotel would be too expensive, especially as she could be here several weeks. There's a lot of paperwork to sort through.' He shoved the suitcase through the gap.

'Let's hope she proves to be competent.'

Calvin hoped so, too. 'How's Mum?'

He phoned his mum every night, but he still needed to know she was okay. As the oldest child, he'd taken on most of the responsibility when his dad had left, unable to bear hearing her crying herself to sleep every night. Although she was in a much better place now, he still felt the need to check on her.

'Your mum's good and sends her love. We had Sunday dinner together yesterday, your sister cooked a lovely roast lamb. Everyone misses you.'

His chest pinched. He missed them, too. His sister was married and worked part-time for a local charity, balancing work with bringing up his twin nieces, and his brother had just finished his physio training.

42

'Hopefully, I'll be back home soon.'

'I doubt that, love.' She headed around to the passenger side.

Frowning, he followed her and opened the door. 'Why do you say that?'

'You can't afford to hire a manager, can you? And unless you free up some of your own money, which I don't think you should do, who else is going to run the place?'

It was a question he'd been asking himself for the past week. Who indeed? Even if he sold his house in Leeds, it would be months before the money came through, and where would he live when he returned home?

'Besides,' she said, patting his chest. 'I think this could be a new start for you. A fresh challenge, something to get your teeth into.'

He experienced another sinking feeling. 'I'm only staying until probate is sorted. Then I'm going back to Leeds.'

She frowned at him. 'And what about the care home?'

'I need to decide whether to sell it, liquidate it or hire a manager to run it.'

Her expression softened. 'I think your uncle Bert envisaged you taking over the running of it.'

'I've no idea why. I'd be rubbish at it.' It still confounded him that his uncle had done that. But then he guessed his uncle was just looking out for him, giving him the option of a second profession after his football career had ended.

She shook her head. 'I think you underestimate yourself.'

'My life's back in Leeds. I have friends there, I want to be close to my family.'

'It's also the scene of the crime,' she said, giving him a sad smile. 'I know you love the place, but do you really want to stay somewhere where you're constantly reminded of all that pain and suffering? You'd never escape it. Wouldn't it be better to make a fresh start somewhere new? Somewhere people don't know you, and where they won't look at you with sadness, but instead see a remarkable and beautiful young man who's making a new life for himself.'

He felt the tears welling up. 'That place isn't Pluckley.'

'No? Shame. It's where I'll be.' And with that, she lowered herself into the car.

Had he heard right? He ducked down to look at her. 'I thought you were only visiting for a few days?'

'I'm not getting any younger, Calvin. It's about time I started looking at care homes, and what better place to move into than the home run by my beloved grandson.'

His heart sank. 'Granny, I'm not staying in Pluckley.'

'So you keep saying.' She patted his hand. 'And you know better than to call me Granny.'

'Sorry… but seriously, this isn't what I want.'

'We'll see. Now, are you going to fetch that last suitcase from the platform before someone pinches it? Only, I'm dying for a cuppa.'

He straightened up, wondering how the hell he was going to fit a third suitcase into his car… and knowing that that was the least of his problems.

Chapter Five

Kate Lawrence stepped onto the deserted railway platform and decided it was the type of night only the dead could enjoy – cold as hell and miserably wet. But this was only to be expected, seeing as she'd just arrived in Kent's most haunted village – something Calvin Johnson had conveniently omitted to mention when he'd offered her a job here.

Amongst the peeling paint and rusted chains holding up the heavy wooden sign, the faded name of Pluckley stared back at her, creaking rhythmically from the rafters, propelled by the occasional swirl of wind that tunnelled through the station. Nice touch. Very eerie.

Zipping up her jacket, she wheeled her suitcase towards the exit.

A single wooden gate led her away from the tracks and onto the station forecourt. The ground was uneven, making manoeuvring her luggage difficult. Still, it wasn't the end of the world: she only had to make it out front, where her client would be waiting for her. A client she'd made the mistake of googling last night – something she'd been regretting ever since.

Her motivation had been driven by uncertainty – after all, she had accepted a job without properly researching the man she'd be working for. He could be an axe murderer for all she knew. Just because he appeared to be nice and kind and sane, with a set of killer dimples and a smile that had rendered her speechless, it didn't mean something darker didn't lurk beneath his attractive exterior. Good-looking men could be jerks, too. She'd been married to one.

What she hadn't expected to find when she'd run a search on his name was that he was a well-known footballer. The image that had popped up on the screen showed him dressed in a smart suit, with his arm around a striking woman with long dark glossy hair and the kind of body that could stop traffic – something which had sent Kate's self-esteem plummeting even further.

She'd slammed her laptop shut, unwilling to read any more details about how successful and talented and gorgeous Calvin Johnson was. She'd learnt all she needed to know. The man was unlikely to be a mass murderer – which alleviated her concerns about his trustworthiness, but only added to the humiliation of having sobbed all over him, the memory of which still made her cringe. It hadn't been her finest moment. Anxiety had a lot to answer for.

On reaching the station forecourt, the sight that greeted her sent her resolve nosediving. A solitary streetlamp shone a weak light on an empty lane, rain-sodden trees and a mass of inky blackness stretching ahead, but no sign of her client.

She checked her phone. The signal was poor and her battery was low. Great.

A sudden gust of wind caught her off balance and she knocked into her suitcase, sending it toppling over. As she bent over to retrieve it, her bag slipped off her shoulder and hit her on the head. The world was conspiring against her. Or rather, Pluckley was.

Having googled Calvin's name, she'd then searched for information about the quaint Kent village, expecting to discover an abundance of fascinating history and images of gorgeous rural cottages. What she hadn't expected to discover was that 'cute' little Pluckley was in fact the epicentre of all things supernatural. Like her life needed any more drama.

Cursing, she grabbed her bag from the floor and shook the mud away. The voice in her head reminded her that she was

46

supposed to stay calm, so she stopped strangling her bag and smoothed back her hair, removing a few rogue strands that'd stuck themselves to her lip gloss. Sucking in a deep breath, she concentrated on breathing. This was not the moment to succumb to another panic attack.

Feeling a fraction calmer, she tapped the screen on her phone, hoping it would spring into life so she could call Calvin and find out where he was, but the battery had died.

Thankfully, help came in the guise of a lone figure walking his dog, visible beneath the solitary streetlamp.

Grabbing her suitcase, she stumbled after him. 'Hello! Excuse me! Can you help me, please?'

The man glanced back, plumes of smoke billowing from his pipe. Unlike her, he was appropriately dressed for the weather in a full-length mac and wellington boots.

'My lift hasn't shown up,' she said, offering him a pleading smile. 'Would you be able to call me a taxi? Only, my phone's died.'

The man looked at her. 'I don't have a mobile.'

'Oh. Is there a taxi rank close by?'

'Ain't no taxis running this time of night. Where d'you need to get to?'

'The Rose Court Care Home. Do you know it?'

His face creased into a frown. 'I do.'

'Is it within walking distance?'

'About a mile or so, I reckon.' He seemed to study her. 'You need to head that way.' He nodded behind her. 'Follow Station Road until you see signs for The Pinnock and then take a left past Screaming Woods. When you reach Devil's Bush, take the lane towards Fright Corner. You'll see the sign for the care home just past the crossroads. You can't miss it – it's by the large oak tree split by lightning.'

Kate wasn't sure whether the man was being genuine, or simply having a laugh at her expense. Either way, it wasn't exactly what she'd wanted to hear. Screaming Woods? Fright Corner? Who came up with these names?

'And I wouldn't hang around,' he said, removing his pipe and whistling for his dog. 'Whatever you see or hear, just keep going.' He patted his dog's head. 'Good luck.'

He wandered off, leaving Kate pondering over his words. *Whatever you see or hear, just keep going?* What on earth did that mean?

But she wouldn't panic; she reminded herself that she was in a remote village in Kent, not a pupil at Hogwarts School. Law of averages dictated that she was unlikely to meet with a sticky end at eight thirty on a Thursday evening at the hands of Moaning Myrtle.

Having suppressed the irrational fear of being bumped off by an irate ghoul, she continued down the lane. So, the place was reputedly haunted. Big deal. It was probably nothing more than a few fanciful old wives' tales that the locals seemed keen to uphold. Clever marketing.

Besides which, she'd discovered a long time ago that people who were alive were a lot more dangerous than people who were already dead. Dead people didn't gamble online, run up debts in your name and impregnate your next-door neighbour.

Her suitcase snagged on a protruding branch, jerking her sideways. Hadn't the local council ever heard of pavements? They were all the rage in civilised towns. Even cute villages like this one had been known to employ twenty-first-century architecture on occasion. But not here. Oh no, the residents of quaint little Pluckley obviously felt it necessary to force its visitors to do battle with the undergrowth.

As she passed the sign for The Pinnock, she guessed she must be heading towards Screaming Woods. A thick blanket of trees loomed either side of the lane, tall and foreboding, and scarily silent. She couldn't work out whether she felt protected by them or entrapped and about to star in her own version of *The Blair Witch Project*.

She continued down the lane, praying the care home wasn't much further; her feet were cold and the damp was starting to creep up her jeans.

The welcome lighting from the railway station had long since dimmed and she was walking in virtual darkness. Only a break in the clouds, allowing a misty shaft of moonlight to penetrate the gloom, indicated the way forwards. A lesser woman would have been intimidated by such a creepy situation. Luckily for her, she was made of sterner stuff – or not, as it transpired.

Her calm resolve was shattered into a frenzy of swearing when the still night air was filled with a loud anguished scream.

She jerked away from the sound, a piercing noise that jabbed at her eardrums. It appeared to be coming from the woods, a weird lingering resonance that echoed around her, freezing her skin as it brushed over her.

She lifted her hands to cover her ears and the noise abruptly stopped. It was replaced by the manic movement of birds, a cacophony of wings beating against the air, as seemingly a whole flock flapped wildly in a bid to escape the terror of the woods.

Ducking away from the noise, she covered her head with her arms, trying to protect herself from the frenzy of birds about to Hitchcock her, but the noise stopped as unexpectedly as it had begun.

Tentatively, she lowered her hands to see what had happened. There was nothing to see. Only an unnatural stillness that shrouded her, as she stood alone in the lane.

With some caution, she peered into the woods, expecting to find the cause of the disturbance. Nothing. No sign of movement, no sound of wings or screaming, or any of the other odd sensations she'd just experienced. What the hell had just happened?

Whatever it was, she wasn't about to hang around for a repeat performance.

Grabbing the handle of her suitcase, she jerked it hard and stumbled onto the road, trying to pick up pace in a bid to get away, but the sound of footsteps stopped her. She spun around, her eyes searching the darkness.

The footsteps neared, accompanied by the sound of ragged breathing. Panic raced through her. Her heart began thumping so hard she could feel it in her teeth. Whoever it was, they were getting closer, advancing as she stood alone in the lane, unprotected and unarmed. Surely she wasn't about to be mugged for a second time?

The distant sound of an approaching vehicle registered with her brain a few moments before a burst of light hurtled around the bend, aiming right at her. Once again, she found herself covering her head with her arms, shielding herself from the blinding glare.

Silhouetted against the shaft of light coming towards her was a man. A man not of this era, but from centuries past: a sword dragging by his side, his demeanour slumped as he staggered towards her, his red frock-coat lit up in the darkness.

She wasn't sure if her scream was audible – the rushing in her ears drowned out any sound, but as the blood drained from her head, she felt herself falling and hit the ground with an almighty thud.

Time seemed to slow as she drifted into a state of semi-consciousness, her body aching from the fall, her mind registering the sound of voices and a car door slamming.

She had no idea how long she lay there shivering, but the next thing she knew, a warm hand was patting her cheek. 'Kate...? Kate, can you hear me?'

Blinking, she opened her eyes to find Calvin Johnson looking down at her. Of course it was him – why was she even surprised?

She'd hoped to regain some of her lost dignity on this trip, and present herself as a competent and level-headed professional, someone reliable and sane, whom he could entrust with his uncle's estate. Instead, she was once again upended, a quivering wreck of a woman with a wet bottom and shaking like a malfunctioning washing machine.

Mortification washed over her. 'I'm not dead, then?'

He bit his lower lip. 'No, not dead. Are you hurt?'

Good question. Was she? She didn't think so. 'I'm fine.'

'Are you sure?'

She wasn't about to admit she had a bruised bum; she was embarrassed enough as it was. 'I'm not hurt, just… wet.' Her jeans were soaked through.

'Can you stand up?' He positioned himself behind her and gently eased her up. 'Lean on me,' he said, holding her steady when she wobbled. 'That's it. You okay?'

'I'm fine.' She blinked a few times, trying to clear her vision, and then she remembered what had just happened. She looked around, but there was no sign of the strange-looking man. Had she imagined it? She rubbed her eyes, wondering if hallucinating was the latest affliction to add to her list of mental health issues.

Calvin had a concerned expression on his face. 'Sorry I wasn't at the station to meet you. One of the care home residents had gone missing, and I had to go and find him.'

Her disgruntlement softened a little. 'That's okay. I probably should've waited at the station and not wandered off, but my phone died and I had no way of contacting you.'

He reached out and removed a twig from her hair. It was a strangely intimate gesture and she wasn't sure whether it was welcome, but he just seemed to be checking she was okay. 'I wondered why you weren't answering your phone. I tried calling to let you know I'd be late.'

She moved away from his touch and removed the rest of the debris herself, trying to regain some composure. 'Did you find the man?'

'I did.' He gave a rueful smile. 'He's going to have a stinking hangover in the morning.' He looked around. 'Where's your luggage?'

As she pointed in the direction of her battered suitcase, a gust of wind whipped through the trees, making the branches rustle. Involuntarily, she jerked away from the noise.

Calvin caught her arm. 'What's wrong?'

'N… nothing,' she said, glancing into the woods, half-expecting to see another apparition, or whatever it was she'd just seen. 'I… I'm fine.'

'Did something spook you?' He sounded concerned.

Forcing a smile, she turned to face him. 'Of course not. I'm fine, really.' What was she supposed to say? *The woods screamed at me and then the Scarlet Pimpernel appeared.* She wouldn't sound delusional at all. 'I'm not used to the quiet, that's all. In London everything is masked by traffic noise. Here you can hear everything, even birds' wings flapping. It's strange.'

'I know what you mean, Leeds is the same. I miss the noise.' He went over to collect her suitcase from the roadside. 'The village is full of strange noises, most of them harmless.'

'Most of them?'

He carried her suitcase over to his car. 'Not worried by a few scary stories, are you?'

'Of course not.' She glanced into the woods one last time, before following him over to the safety of the vehicle. He obviously hadn't seen the strange man in the red coat, so she wasn't going to mention it – he'd think she was nuts. Even more nuts than he probably already suspected. And that was the last thing she needed – he might rethink his decision to employ her.

Having loaded her suitcase into the boot of his sporty Mazda, he opened the passenger door. 'After you.'

'I'm all wet and muddy,' she said, staring at the pristine upholstery. 'I'll mess up your fancy car.'

'It'll wash off,' he said, shrugging. 'Don't worry about it.'

Shrugging off her jacket, she turned it inside out and placed it over the seat. 'All the same, I'd rather not make a mess.'

He waited until she was buckled in before closing the door and heading around to the driver's side. Her new client might unnerve her, but she'd rather be trapped inside a vehicle with him than endure another moment dealing with the spooky elements of Pluckley. And she'd thought country life would be relaxing?

He climbed in beside her and started the engine. 'How was your journey?'

'Good, thanks.' She risked a glance at him as the interior light faded. He was just as impressive as she remembered. His hair was tied up, exposing the shaved section underneath, and his expensive watch glinted in the light, the chunky metal strap poking out from beneath the sleeve of his Abercrombie & Fitch hoodie. He matched the car – sleek, sporty and powerful.

If Calvin Johnson was the high-end version of cars, she was a fairground dodgem, with poor steering, fading paintwork and suffering from one too many crashes.

Shoving the vehicle into gear, he drove off at such speed, she instinctively reached out to grab the handle. When a bowing tree branch smacked against the window, she ducked.

He glanced over. 'Am I driving too fast?'

'It's fine,' she lied, unwilling to admit to her aversion to speed, along with her other foibles. She was already feeling enough of a flake as it was.

'Sorry, it's a bad habit of mine,' he said, slowing down. 'My granny's always telling me off for driving too fast.'

For some reason this surprised her. It seemed odd for such a successful man to be worried about what an elderly relative thought about his driving.

True to his word, he slowed to a gentler speed and continued along the dark lanes, without causing her belly to flip. She was grateful.

'I wasn't sure whether you would've eaten,' he said, decelerating when a sharp bend came into view. 'I asked our chef, Geraldine, to make you something. I hope soup's okay. It's in the microwave, ready to be warmed up.'

Kate's stomach rumbled. She hadn't eaten tonight, mainly because her appetite hadn't been great of late, but the idea of home-made soup definitely appealed. 'That's kind of her, I hope it wasn't too much trouble.'

'She was happy to help,' he said, with a shrug. 'I've made up a room for you. It can be a bit chilly in the home, as the

53

windows aren't double-glazed, but I lit the fire before I left, so the room should be warm when you arrive.'

Surely he hadn't made up the room himself? He'd probably instructed the housekeeping staff to do it. She couldn't imagine him tucking in bedsheets and wrestling with a duvet cover – he didn't seem the type. Still, it was nice of him to light a fire for her. 'You didn't have to go to so much effort. I'm here to work, not have a holiday.'

'You need to be comfy, especially as you'll be here a while. Besides, I don't want you changing your mind and leaving me.' He glanced over. 'I need you.'

'I need you, too,' she said instinctively, before cringing with embarrassment. 'Sorry… I mean, well… you know… professionally.'

A brief smile tugged at his lips. 'I know what you meant.'

He returned to concentrating on driving. She was glad. Interactions with Calvin Johnson had an unnerving effect on her.

Now that they were travelling at a sensible speed, she was able to relax and enjoy the warmth from the car heater circling her legs. She looked out of the window, watching the damp smearing against the glass, and listened to the hypnotic swish of the windscreen wipers.

As they drove through the narrow twisted lanes, an imposing church spire came into view above the treetops. Further down the road they hit a fork with a set of wooden signs that signalled left for Devil's Bush and straight ahead for Fright Corner. The dog walker hadn't been making up the names, then.

'This is where they had a bad lightning strike,' Calvin said, pointing to where a massive, blackened oak tree loomed ahead.

The sky suddenly lit up with a flash of lightning and she could see a big split running down the middle of the trunk. It was a wonder the thing was still standing, but as she'd already discovered, the dead liked to reside in Pluckley.

They drove through a set of large, rusted iron gates, the pillars either side surmounted by gargoyles. It was a moment before the care home came into view. When it did, she feared the onset of another panic attack.

As they pulled up, she stared out the window, hoping the sight might soften on further inspection.

Gingerly, she climbed out, gazing up at the ornate gothic construction, with its multitude of grey stone walls and rectangular windows silhouetted against the darkening November skyline.

Another crackle of lightning split the smouldering clouds above, connecting with the top of an east-facing turret. The Rose Court Care Home wouldn't look out of place in a *Hammer House of Horror* production.

Another deep rumble of thunder rolled across the sky.

Jesus, this place was creepy. *What next?* Vincent Price laughter? Dracula flapping the reins of a horse-drawn hearse? She had to question whether working here was really going to solve her problems, or instead send her resolve plummeting into further despair.

Calvin appeared next to her with her suitcase. 'Head inside, the door's unlocked. There's something I need to do first.'

'Sure,' she said. It wasn't like anything else had been normal so far tonight.

Dragging her suitcase up to the wooden door, she glanced back and watched Calvin jog back to his car, his gait athletic and effortless. He didn't seem to fit in with this place any more than she did. It was certainly a strange place for a famous footballer to be residing, even if it was only temporarily, while he dealt with his uncle's estate. She would have thought he'd be staying in a nearby five-star resort with spa facilities and a gym. Maybe there weren't any in this part of the world.

As she watched him, a man's face suddenly appeared at the back window of the Mazda. It gave her such a jolt that she screamed and jumped backwards. Her ankle buckled under her and, for the second time that evening, she found herself landing on her bum.

Calvin came racing over. 'Are you okay? What happened?'

She waved a finger at the face, recognising the red coat and the wild black hair. 'Who... who's that man?'

He looked over to where she was pointing. 'Oh, that's Rowan Blakely, the care home resident that went missing tonight.' He took her hands and pulled her to her feet. 'Are you okay?' His soft Yorkshire accent was at odds with the panic racing through her.

No, she was not okay. But as Calvin seemed completely unperturbed by the sight of a gruesome creature sitting in his vehicle − face twisted with pain, eyes crazed and searching − who was she to comment. 'Why is he dressed like that?'

'Rowan gives talks at the local pub, he's an expert on the ghosts of Pluckley. He had a bit too much to drink tonight, so the landlord called me and asked me to pick him up. By the time I got there, Rowan had gone walkabout. I found him staggering down the lane where I picked you up.'

'Right.' So it hadn't been a ghost then − it was a real person. She could relax, she wasn't going crazy... if you ignored the strange noises and birds flapping manically in the woods.

Calvin opened the front door for her. 'Welcome to Pluckley.'

Welcome, indeed.

Chapter Six

Friday, 26th November

It was gone eight a.m. by the time Calvin headed upstairs to check on Kate. He hadn't had the best start to the day and was running late. Geraldine's hip was playing up, so he'd offered to take Suki for a walk, intending to combine exercising the dog with his morning run. He'd envisaged jogging through Screaming Woods with the dog obediently trotting behind him. Instead, the damn creature kept stopping to sniff, pee and dig up random pieces of wood. All this was followed by rolling in several muddy puddles and then disappearing into the forest like a blonde bullet, when she'd picked up the scent of another animal.

What had started out as a low-impact jog turned into a full-on sprint as he tried to keep track of her. He could only imagine the grief he'd get from Geraldine if he lost her precious dog, or his heart consultant at his next check-up when they reviewed the data from the implantable loop recorder inserted in his chest. He'd religiously stuck to his permitted exercise regime since being diagnosed, but the structured plan drawn up for him hadn't taken into account the unpredictability of chasing after a blessed dog.

By the time they arrived back at the care home, they were both covered in mud, soaking wet and in desperate need of a bath.

Tying up his damp hair, he pulled on his green Nike hoodie and climbed the stairs to the second floor. The top floor was reserved for the staff team, and it was where they stored all the linens, drugs and medical equipment. The first floor was the nursing floor, where the residents slept, and the ground floor was the communal area, where the kitchen, dining room and living room were. It was also where his room was situated.

His late uncle had lived on site when he'd been manager and had converted a section of the east wing into a self-contained apartment, consisting of a snug bedroom and a living room with an open fire and a huge bay window. It was rustic and draughty, and a far cry from the plush hotels he'd stayed in as a footballer, but it didn't bother him.

After all, it was only temporary. He'd be back home in Leeds soon, enjoying the comfort of his new-build house, with its latest gadgets and stark white decor – something Ainsley had insisted on. He could only imagine her reaction if she saw where he was living now. Not that she'd care. And besides, maybe he preferred period and rustic to magazine contemporary. It was certainly less clinical. All that white had strained his eyes.

Punching in the security code, he let himself into the staff area, which appeared to be deserted. It wasn't surprising. The residents would have been washed and dressed by now, and would be eating breakfast, either in their rooms or downstairs in the dining room. The staff would be administering medications and doing their nursing rounds.

He hadn't seen Kate in the dining room or in the library, so he assumed she was still in her room. He wasn't sure whether knocking on her bedroom door was appropriate, but after last night it seemed wrong not to check on her. She hadn't seemed overly enamoured with Pluckley. Her nervous state hadn't been helped by the stormy weather or being left stranded at the train station. Encountering Rowan Blakely dressed in his period costume had been the final straw and he'd feared she was about to have another panic attack.

He'd become accustomed to the weird noises and strange behaviours of the village, but Kate hadn't had the opportunity to adjust. She was probably hiding under the covers, shivering and questioning her decision to work here. Or worse, she'd already packed up and left.

He tapped on her door. 'Hello…? Kate…? Are you up yet?'

No answer.

The door was ajar and he could see that the room was flooded with daylight, which meant she must be awake. He tried again, knocking harder this time and causing the door to swing open. 'Kate, are you in here?'

There was no sign of her. Her suitcase was lying on the seat by the window, so he figured she hadn't run off, which was something.

Closing the door, he backtracked down the corridor and jogged down to the first floor, in case she'd got lost and had ended up in the wrong place. There were ten bedrooms in total, but currently only four were occupied.

After his uncle's death, Hanna had made the decision not to accept any new residents until the future of the care home had been decided, which was fair enough, especially as they were running on a reduced staff team. This just left Rowan Blakely, Larry Redding, and Deshad and Priya Bakshi in residence.

He heard Kate's voice before he saw her; she was in Priya's room.

Pausing by the doorway, he glanced in, surprised to see Kate handing Priya's husband a cup of tea. 'I hope it's not too strong,' she said, holding it until he had a firm grip.

'I take it as it comes,' Deshad said, smiling.

'Everything okay in here?' Calvin asked from the doorway, puzzled as to what was happening.

She startled at the sound of his voice. She was wearing a formal grey business suit, with a pale blue shirt underneath. Her fair hair was tied up and secured by a clip. It was a complete contrast to how she'd looked last night, all dishevelled and… damp.

'Morning,' she said, offering him a shaky smile. 'I got lost trying to find the library and ended up on the wrong floor.'

'Where's Natalie?'

'I don't know who Natalie is,' she said, looking self-conscious. 'This gentleman asked for a cup of tea, and as no one was around, I thought I'd get him one. I'd seen the kitchenette at the end of the hallway, so it was no bother.' She hesitated, as if realising she might have done something wrong. 'Have I overstepped?'

Guilt nudged him in the ribs. 'Of course not, it's kind of you to help out. I'm just wondering why Natalie isn't here. She's our night nurse and usually sorts out breakfast before she finishes her shift.' He came into the room. 'Morning, Deshad. Has Priya been washed this morning?'

'Not yet,' he replied, cradling his tea. 'It's not a problem – we're happy to wait. Natalie's probably dealing with Jacob. Poor girl was in here several times last night turning Priya and she's probably exhausted. Please don't be angry with her.'

Calvin wasn't angry; he was concerned. He knew it was a tough ask looking after the residents with only two nurses, even though both Rowan and Lucky Larry were still active and mobile. But Priya's stroke had left the fifty-five-year-old unable to manage the most basic tasks and this presented the team with a number of additional challenges, especially as she had lost the ability to communicate.

He was about to go in search of Natalie when she rushed into the room, holding a screaming Jacob. 'I'm so sorry! Jacob threw up everywhere and I had to change my uniform. He refused to settle and I've been playing catch-up all night.'

The pair of them looked exhausted, and once again Calvin felt overwhelmed with guilt. Natalie's pale skin seemed almost see-through this morning and her dark red hair was shoved into a lopsided ponytail.

'It's fine, Natalie. Don't worry. Is Jacob sick? Does he need to see a doctor?'

'I don't think so.' She touched his forehead. 'He hasn't got a temperature, he's just grumpy. Can you take him while I sort out Priya?'

The baby was dumped into his arms. 'Sure. No problem.'

Jacob was heavier than he'd expected and he had to adjust his grip to settle the kid against his chest. He was used to handling babies; he'd been very hands-on with his twin nieces and instinctively began rocking Jacob, hoping to quell his screaming.

Natalie went over to Priya. 'Good morning, my love. Let's get you washed and dressed, shall we? It's always nice to be in fresh clothes.'

It never ceased to amaze him how kind the staff were to the residents, showing genuine concern over their wellbeing. They certainly weren't in the profession for the money, of that he was certain.

'We'll wait outside,' he said, gesturing for Kate to follow him into the corridor.

Deshad acted as Priya's full-time carer, which was just as well, as they'd struggle to cope with her needs if he wasn't on hand 24/7 to help them. Following his wife's stroke, Deshad had given up work to care for her, and when Priya had deteriorated and moved into the care home, he had moved in with her. A situation Calvin's late uncle had agreed to and supported.

Unfortunately, the local authority would only pay for Priya's care needs, so Deshad was living with them rent-free. Calvin had no issue with this, as he knew how desperate the couple were to stay together. But he wasn't so sure whether any new management would see it the same way, which was something else that was playing on his mind and impeding his decision about the care home's future.

'Have you had breakfast?' he asked Kate, as she closed the bedroom door behind her. Her shirt had become untucked and she was unsteady on her heels.

'I'm not hungry,' she said, inspecting the empty corridor. 'You don't seem to have many staff working this morning. Is that usual?'

He let out a sigh. 'It shouldn't be, but we don't have the money to pay the staff we do have, let alone recruit new people. It's not ideal, I know.' He bounced Jacob in his arms, grateful that his efforts seemed to be working: the screaming had softened to a disgruntled whimper.

'When were they last paid?' she asked, suddenly seeming to notice her dishevelled state. Tutting, she straightened her jacket, her cheeks colouring slightly.

She was cute when she blushed. He glanced away, embarrassed at where his thoughts had been headed. 'Six months ago.'

'It's a wonder they've stayed,' she said, tucking in her shirt.

'Tell me about it.' It was something that was giving him sleepless nights. So much so, he'd contacted his financial adviser and asked him to sell shares for two of his investments. Something his adviser had urged him against doing, reminding him that he might need the money further down the line if his health deteriorated, but that wasn't enough to dissuade him. His conscience wouldn't allow him to sit back and watch the situation at the care home continue to deteriorate any longer.

The door at the end of the corridor swung open and Hanna appeared, her jet-black hair a contrast to the magnolia decor. 'Where's Natalie?' she barked, marching towards him like she was accusing him of abducting the woman. 'Breakfast tray for Deshad and Priya still in kitchen. Why?'

'Natalie's running behind this morning,' he said, afraid Hanna's abrupt voice might set Jacob off screaming again. 'She's with Priya now, washing and dressing her.'

Hanna made a point of checking the watch attached to her nurse's tunic. 'This late? Priya need medication. She need food first.'

Calvin hated confrontation, especially in front of an audience. He didn't like the idea of Kate Lawrence discovering the depths of his management inadequacies. Although why, he wasn't sure – it wasn't like she wasn't battling demons of her own. 'Can you bring up the breakfast tray for her, Hanna?'

Hanna looked incredulous. 'I have enough to do. Now you want me to take on extra duties?' Her hands went to her hips, the veins in the shaved section of her head pulsating with anger.

He nodded at Jacob as if to say, *we're all having to take on extra duties*. 'Just this once. I'd really appreciate it.'

'I can fetch the breakfast tray,' Kate cut in, her eyes darting between them. 'I know where the kitchen is, I had supper there last night.'

Calvin turned to her. 'You don't have to do that, it's not your responsibility.'

'Not my responsibility either,' snapped Hanna. 'But you happy to ask me. Who is this woman anyway?'

Calvin cringed at Hanna's rudeness. 'This is Kate Lawrence, the solicitor helping us apply for probate. She's here to help, okay?' He glared at her, hoping his expression warned her to 'be nice'.

Hanna made a harrumphing noise. 'About time. Care home going to the dogs.'

He closed his eyes, wishing he could wave a magic wand and disappear somewhere. This was not how he'd imagined his life to be. He was not equipped to deal with this.

'Really, let me do it,' Kate said, seemingly unperturbed by the frostiness of the head nurse. 'It's no bother, it'll take me two minutes. The stairs are this way, right?' She pointed to where Hanna had appeared moments earlier, already edging towards the door, as if eager to escape. He couldn't blame her.

'Turn right at the bottom,' he called after her, as she reached the doorway. 'The kitchen's across the hallway. Thanks, Kate. I owe you.'

'Not a problem. Back soon.'

When she'd disappeared from view, he turned to find Hanna glaring at him. 'Not acceptable,' she said, jabbing a finger at him. 'Bad management.'

'I know, and I'm sorry. But I'm in the process of freeing up funds so I can pay the staff and arrange extra help. I promise to get this sorted, Hanna.'

'You'd better,' she said, storming off. 'Losing patience.'

Calvin stood in the hallway, his stomach weighed down by guilt and frustration. Like his confidence hadn't been dented enough these last few months. He'd lost his career, his girlfriend, and now he was making a mess of dealing with his uncle's affairs.

He hated letting everyone down. Maybe it would be better if he just used the money he was freeing up to hire a new manager and walk away from the whole thing. But what would happen to the staff and residents? Would the new manager allow Deshad to stay on rent-free? Would they show sympathy towards Natalie's situation? Tolerance for Hanna's temper? And what about his granny? Could he really walk away from her within days of her arrival?

Jacob made a gurgling sound and Calvin realised the baby had stopped crying. Looking down, he was met with a pair of sleepy blue eyes gazing up at him. Calvin cradled him closer and watched as his eyes drifted shut. The fidgeting stopped, the hands lowered and Jacob became a cosy weight in his arms.

He'd always liked kids. Being invited to clubs and schools to talk about his career had always been fun. Not so much the standing up and talking bit – he'd never been comfortable doing that – but the sessions usually ended with a game of football, him against thirty or so kids, all chasing after the ball, tying to tackle him and making him laugh with their enthusiasm.

He'd been proud to be the face of a local kids' charity, encouraging youngsters into sport, and he was patron of his youth team, Wortley Football Club. He'd even envisaged having kids himself one day, mini footballers that he could coach and encourage. But that seemed like another shattered dream and unlikely to happen anytime soon.

He sucked in a breath, trying to ease the ache in his chest that had nothing to do with his HCM.

A bang further down the corridor alerted him to Kate reversing through the doorway, carrying the tea tray. Her suit jacket had popped open and a few strands of hair had escaped from her hair clip. She wobbled on her high heels as she walked towards him, trying not to spill anything.

'I would offer to help, but I have my hands full.'

Her focus remained on the tea tray. 'That's okay, at least he's stopped crying. Is he asleep?'

'Out like a light.'

'You've obviously got the knack.' She stopped by Priya's door. 'Shall I knock?'

'It's better to wait. Natalie will be out when she's done. We try to preserve the residents' dignity where possible, by not intruding unless absolutely necessary.'

'Fair enough.' She lowered the tea tray to the floor. 'I guess it's not nice having to rely on others to look after you.'

'I'd hate it.'

'God, me too,' she said, stifling a yawn. When she stood up, she bumped against the wall, causing her foot to slip out of her shoe. Blowing a strand of hair away from her face, she smoothed down her skirt and adjusted her footwear. She looked uncomfortable, like she was in constant battle with her clothes.

He gently swayed Jacob, praying he would stay asleep. 'Did you sleep okay?'

'Not really, the windows kept banging open. I got up a few times to close them, but gave up in the end and left them open. The strangest thing, though: this morning, when I woke up, they were closed. I don't remember shutting them, but I must've done. That, or it was the wind.'

'Bound to be,' he said, hoping she didn't mention these strange goings-on to Rowan, who would offer a completely different explanation for windows randomly opening in the night. Not that Calvin believed in ghosts himself, even if he did feel haunted by recent events.

Priya's door opened. 'All done,' Natalie said, heading over to Calvin. 'He's asleep? How did you do that?'

'Luck,' he said, handing over a sleeping Jacob. 'I'd take the chance to grab some sleep yourself while you can, before he wakes up.'

Natalie kissed her son's cheek. 'I should really carry on working, I have another hour to make up.'

'Don't be daft. Clock off and rest up. You need it.' He wondered whether it would be tactless to tell her how exhausted she looked. 'I'll see to Deshad and Priya's breakfast.'

Natalie looked relieved. 'Thanks.' Cradling Jacob, she turned to Kate. 'I'm Natalie, by the way. Calvin mentioned you were arriving today.'

'Nice to meet you.' Kate bent down to pick up the tea tray.

'Here, let me.' Calvin took the tray from her. 'Thanks again for fetching it.' His hand brushed hers and he was shocked by how cold she was.

Kate gave him a half-smile. 'Happy to help.'

'Give me a minute and I'll show you where the library is.'

Leaving Kate and Natalie in the corridor, Calvin delivered the tea tray. He offered to feed Priya, but he knew Deshad wanted to be the one caring for his wife, so he left the man to it. It was a testament to his love that every day he carefully spoon-fed Priya, read to her and held her hand while they watched TV. His eyes would be fixed on the screen; hers would be gazing up at the ceiling, lost and unfocused. It was so tragic that their love affair had been cruelly interrupted, and incredibly sad that Deshad's life had been affected as much as his wife's. It was no way to live, for either of them.

Kate was alone in the corridor when he returned. 'Natalie's gone for a lie-down,' she said, tucking a loose strand of hair behind her ear. 'She said thanks again for letting her finish early.'

'I'd hardly call it finishing early. She works too many hours as it is.'

'Then the quicker we apply for probate, the better.'

'Agreed. The library's this way.' He glanced back, noticing how Kate's feet continually slipped out of her shoes when she walked. 'I'm sorry about Hanna – she can be a bit abrupt at times.'

'I imagine she's stressed.'

'She feels let down, and I can't blame her for venting. But that's no excuse for being rude to you. You didn't deserve that.'

'Don't worry about me,' Kate said, as they reached the doorway. 'It's a testing time for everyone. I just hope I can make quick progress on dealing with the estate. I'm sure I'd feel just as aggrieved if I was in her situation.' And then she flinched, before looking flustered. 'Not that I'm blaming you. I know this isn't your fault.'

'But I'm the one who needs to sort it out,' he said, holding the door open for her. 'The library's on the ground floor.' He waited until she was through the door before leading her downstairs into the large hallway. 'Over there is the dining room.' He pointed to where Geraldine was clearing away the breakfast things. 'Next door is the activities room, and over here is the lounge and library.' He opened the door. 'After you.'

Kate faltered almost as soon as she entered the room. 'Oh, wow, look at all these books.' She walked around, her face tilted upwards as her eyes scanned the floor-to-ceiling bookcases, all crammed full of publications, sealed behind glass-fronted doors. 'Talk about impressive.'

'Dusty, too,' he said, following her into the room and noticing the drop in temperature. 'I don't think it's been properly cleaned since my great-uncle died.'

She turned slowly, taking in the carved wooden door surrounds and large oil paintings hanging on the wall above the fireplace. 'Hardly seems fair to pay for a cleaner when you can't pay the staff.'

'Exactly.' He wiped away a sheen of dust from the mantlepiece. 'Hanna and Natalie clean the residents' floor themselves, and Geraldine does the kitchen, but the other areas have been a bit neglected of late. I try to do them myself when I can, but other, more urgent, stuff keeps coming up.'

She turned to him. 'I can't imagine you cleaning. You look too… you know, pristine.' Her eyes travelled over his designer sportswear – not disapprovingly, but he felt uncomfortable just the same.

'I'm not precious about getting my hands dirty,' he said, feeling defensive at the implication that he was above such

67

things. He'd done a lot of cleaning in his time. You had to when you were part of a single-parent family – it was all hands on deck. 'Talking of clothes—'

'I know, I know, I'm sorry.' She held up her hands. 'I look a right mess – you don't have to tell me. I'll tidy myself up.' She rebuttoned her jacket again.

He smiled at her reaction. 'I was going to say, don't feel like you have to wear a suit on my account. Wear whatever you feel comfortable in. I'd rather you be warm than worry about getting mucky.'

She raised an eyebrow. 'Are you sure?'

'Absolutely. This isn't a London law office.' He glanced at the stained ceiling and scuffed wooden floorboards. 'It's a rundown period building. You can wear a bunny onesie if you want.'

She surprised him by laughing. 'I wish I'd packed it now.'

He wasn't sure whether she was joking. 'I didn't get around to lighting the fire this morning, I got held up. Sorry about that, it's a bit chilly in here. I'll light it before I leave.' He gestured to the large open fire, with its stone surround. 'I've cleared out my late uncle's desk and given it a wipe, so I hope it's okay for you to use. There's Wi-Fi, but no phone in here. The mobile signal's patchy, but it improves if you head towards the rear of the building.'

'I'm sure it'll be fine,' she said, nodding towards the desk. 'It's a beautiful piece of furniture. Is it a Chippendale?'

'If it is, then we'll be selling it.'

She smiled. 'I'll add it to the asset register.' She went over to the window and knelt on the padded seat nestled inside the large bay alcove. As she leant forwards to gaze out of the window, her bum strained against the material of her skirt and he quickly looked away. 'This window is amazing,' she said, peering outside. 'It lets in so much light.'

'Lets in a lot of cold, too. I think the lead needs replacing.'

'Where are the ledgers?'

'Over here.' He pointed to the shelving next to the fireplace. 'They're roughly in date order, filed in decades. The oldest ones are at the top.'

He watched her almost topple backwards and she strained to see the top shelf.

'You'll need this,' he said, gesturing to the giant set of stepladders on casters. 'It looks like a deathtrap, but it's pretty sturdy. It holds my weight.'

'If I'm going up and down that thing all day, then you're probably right: maybe a suit and heels aren't the best option.'

The library door creaked open and Esme appeared. 'Ah, here you are,' she said, looking smartly turned out in a blue blazer. 'Geraldine said you'd arrived safely. I'm Esme.'

'Kate Lawrence.' Kate shook Esme's hand. 'Are you a resident here?'

'Yes,' she said, at the same time Calvin said, 'No.'

Kate looked between them.

'Esme is my grandmother,' he said, incurring a look of wrath from his granny. 'My late uncle's sister-in-law. She's visiting for a few days to help me sort out the estate.'

Granny Esme fixed him with her steely gaze, but he didn't give her the satisfaction of returning her look. After a few seconds, she turned to Kate, her gaze softening. 'I know quite a bit about my late brother-in-law's affairs, so please ask me anything you're not sure about.'

Kate smiled. 'Thanks, I will.'

Esme fixed her grandson with a look. 'How do you expect this young lady to work in such a cold room, Calvin? Light the fire, for goodness' sake.'

He supressed the urge to roll his eyes. 'I'll do it now.'

'And while the room heats up, Kate and I will head to the kitchen for some breakfast. I've asked Geraldine to make some of her delicious pancakes.'

'Oh, I'm not hungry,' Kate said, looking embarrassed. 'I'd rather just start work. There's a lot to do.'

But Esme wasn't to be deterred. 'Geraldine tells me you haven't eaten this morning.'

Kate glanced at Calvin, as if looking for an ally. 'Like I said, I'm not hungry.'

'You cannot possibly work on an empty stomach, I won't hear of it. Come with me, my dear.' Esme hooked her arm through Kate's and led her over to the door. 'Besides, I'm keen to hear all about you. Calvin tells me you're currently unemployed?'

Kate glanced back at Calvin, her eyes wide as if to say, 'Help me!'

'Sorry,' he mouthed, feeling bad for her, but knowing better than to overrule his grandmother.

Kate didn't look happy. He wasn't overly happy himself.

Chapter Seven

Tuesday, 30th November

When the stepladder shifted beneath her and threatened to topple her off for the third time that morning, Kate grabbed hold of the bookcase, trying to regain her balance. Why did the stupid thing keep moving? One moment she was reaching up for another ledger, the next she was sliding across the floor, suspended in mid-air and clinging on for dear life. It was like the wretched thing had a mind of its own.

When she was sure the ladder had stopped moving, she tentatively began her descent, edging down one step at a time, ensuring her foot connected with each rung before letting go. With the 1956 ledger squashed between her and the rungs, it wouldn't take much to topple her off. Cataloguing the list of assets was slow going. She'd been at it for three days and had only covered two years so far. At this rate it would take her months to complete the task of logging all of Bertram Williams's estate. That was, assuming she lived long enough to complete the job, since the library seemed to be conspiring against her.

Easing herself onto solid ground, she was relieved to have survived another trip up the stepladder. If it wasn't the ladder moving of its own accord, it was the lights randomly flickering, or the window suddenly swinging inwards and banging against the wall, making her jump. And don't get her started on the open fire, which either refused to stay lit or burst into a flurry of flames for no apparent reason. Working at The Rose Court Care Home was both unnerving and exhausting.

It wasn't like she was sleeping much, either. Noises in the middle of the night kept jolting her awake. Whether it was doors slamming, water pipes rattling or the wind howling down the chimney shaft, it was impossible to settle. And she'd thought London was noisy?

Carrying the ledger over to the desk, she wiped the cover with a damp cloth. Calvin had been right: working in the library was a filthy job. It was cold, too. She hadn't needed telling twice about her clothing and had discarded her suits for fleece-lined boots, thick leggings and warm woollen tops that covered her bum.

It had been an odd few days, to say the least. Aside from the strange living environment, she felt like she was working for an eclectic group of people who might one day star in the board game Cluedo. Geraldine could regularly be heard dissecting a large slab of meat with a cleaver; Natalie would appear like a spirit in the dead of night, carrying a metal tray that contained various lethal-looking syringes; and Hanna could rival Nurse Ratched when it came to her bedside manner.

Which just left Calvin, who – like her – also appeared to be out of his comfort zone. She almost felt sorry for him, as he desperately tried to keep the peace and prevent any blood spillage. But then she remembered he was here temporarily and would soon be back living his best life, earning millions from elite sport and socialising with gorgeous models. He didn't need her sympathy.

Aside from the worry for the care-home problems, which to be fair, Calvin had prewarned her about, a small part of her had actually relaxed over the last few days. Which was a puzzle in itself, and probably said a lot about her mental state. Perhaps it was the change of scenery, or no longer fearing the arrival of bailiffs or red demand letters dropping onto the doormat. Whatever it was, the knot in her stomach had finally started to loosen. She'd even managed to read a few chapters of her romance saga last night, before dropping off to sleep – something she hadn't done for ages. Of course, she'd woken soon after, when the window had banged open, but feeling relaxed enough to read in the first place had felt like a breakthrough.

Picking up the card her mum had sent her, she read the message again.

Good luck with the new job, Katiekins!

The use of her childhood nickname brought a lump to her throat. Her mum had even enclosed a small Advent calendar. Kate positioned it above the desk, ready to begin opening the little windows tomorrow.

The last few Christmases had been a sad and lonely occasion, a reminder of all that she'd lost. But it was a time of year she used to love, so a part of her still hoped that maybe one day her future Christmases might not be so grim. A girl could hope.

She was about to continue searching for further dormant accounts, when her phone rang. It was her cousin, Beth.

'Am I glad to hear from you,' Kate said, making a detour over to the window seat to enjoy the view. The morning frost had yet to thaw and the trees sparkled in the sunlight. 'I think I might've bitten off more than I can handle.'

'I could've told you that.' Beth sounded amused. 'This commission had disaster written all over it. What's happened?'

'I hadn't considered the number of distractions I'd have to contend with. I knew dealing with the estate was going to be challenging, but I thought relocating here was meant to make life easier, not harder.'

'How so?'

Kate checked the door was closed so she wouldn't be overheard. 'For a start, the chef keeps force-feeding me. The care team want to know when they're going to get paid, and Calvin's grandmother is determined to uncover my entire backstory. I feel like I'm being vetted. For what, I've no idea. Maybe she's worried I'm going to run off with the family silver.'

Beth laughed. 'She's probably sussing out whether you're a suitable match for her grandson.'

Kate almost slid off the window seat. 'Hardly.'

'Why not? You said he was good-looking.'

'He is, but he's way out of my league. Besides, he has a girlfriend – a very hot girlfriend. And anyway, romance is the last thing on my mind.'

'Who said anything about romance? No-strings sex on the other hand… now that might do you the power of good.'

'Or finish me off completely.' She leant back against the window, jolting forwards when the cold seeped through her cardigan. 'I'm sticking to my plan of sorting my life out with no distractions.' The idea of getting involved with anyone made her shiver, and not in a good way. She'd had her fill of men.

'No reason why you can't enjoy a bit of harmless fun in the meantime. And what do you mean, he's out of your league? Stop putting yourself down. You're a catch. Any man would be lucky to snag you.'

'Snag me? Jesus, Beth, I'm not a fish.' If she expected a sarcastic comeback, it didn't materialise, and instead she was met with stony silence. 'Beth…? Are you there?'

The blessed phone signal had died.

Shuffling off the seat, Kate walked around the room, hoping the little bar would reappear on her screen. 'Beth…? Can you hear me?'

'…You… need to… get back… out there…'

'Hang on, I can't hear you properly.' Kate lifted the phone, turning it in different directions, but it made no difference. She headed to the far side of the room, remembering what Calvin had said about the signal improving at the rear of the building. 'Is that better?'

'…Can't… deny… yourself… rest… of… your life…'

Kate noticed a door she hadn't been through before, at the back of the room. She assumed it linked the library with the communal lounge area. Maybe the signal would be better in there.

Turning the handle, she pushed open the door. Only, it wasn't the lounge: it was a cosy living space, with an archway leading through to a bedroom. The lights were on, revealing an unmade rumpled bed with clothes strewn across it.

Common sense told her someone lived here – someone who was in the process of getting dressed. She needed to retreat, and quickly. But before she could move, the bathroom door opened and Calvin Johnson appeared... naked.

Every nerve ending in her body screamed at her to run. Close her eyes, turn away and leave immediately. She was intruding, invading his privacy. Her presence in his private bedroom was wholly inappropriate and mortifying. She needed to leave... now.

Unfortunately, the message didn't seem to be getting through to her feet. They remained glued to the spot. Her mouth had dropped open, and her eyes were wide and unblinking, fixated on the sight ahead. Calvin Johnson, wet from the shower, naked and... and very... naked. Had she mentioned he was *naked*?

In contrast to the abundance of hair on his head, his body was completely smooth, apart from his clipped goatee, but she wasn't looking at that. She was staring at his bare chest, paler than the rest of him, each rib and muscle defined as if it had been sculptured. The tattoos on his arms travelled upwards and dipped over the curve of his shoulders, which in turn led her eyes downwards to where his waist narrowed, leading to his slim hips and...

'Shit!' He'd spotted her.

The shock of getting sprung broke the spell and she recoiled. 'Oh, my God, I'm so sorry,' she blurted, averting her gaze.

'What the hell?' He grabbed a towel off the bed and wrapped it around his midriff.

'I had no idea this was your room,' she said, stumbling backwards. 'I was trying to get a better signal.' She lifted her phone as evidence, trying desperately to justify her intrusion, aware of her cousin's faint voice at the other end asking, 'What's going on?'

75

'I'm not dressed,' he said, stating the obvious and looking self-conscious… although he had absolutely no reason to be. It was like he'd been airbrushed. That was beside the point. She was encroaching. Worse, she'd openly gawped. The fact that he was gorgeous was irrelevant. He was entitled to undress in the safety of his own room without an audience.

'I'm really sorry,' she repeated for the umpteenth time, turning and smacking her hip against the corner of a wooden dresser. 'Pretend I was never here.' Like that was going to happen… for her, anyway. The image of his body was singed into her brain. Scalded onto her eyeballs. It wasn't something she was likely to forget. Ever.

She rushed from the room, aware that her face was burning hot and her hands were clammy. It said something about the state of her pathetic love-life that the mere sight of a naked body could evoke such a reaction. They were work colleagues. He was her employer, for crying out loud. They weren't even friends. She wasn't sure whether that made it worse, or better. Either way, nothing about their arrangement required them to see each other naked. She'd crossed a line – however unintentionally.

Thankfully, Geraldine wasn't in the kitchen, so Kate was able to escape unseen via the back door and hide around the rear of the building. Resting her hands on her knees, she sucked in a few deep breaths, trying to stem the onslaught of another panic attack. Hyperventilating over a man was not cool. She needed to get a grip. Her heart was racing so fast, it was a wonder it hadn't combusted.

It was a good few seconds before she was able to lift the phone to her ear. 'Are you still there?' She leant against the wall, trying to catch her breath.

'What the hell's going on?' Beth sounded concerned. 'Why did you scream?'

Kate straightened. 'I screamed?'

'Like you'd seen a dead body.'

Oh, hell. Kate closed her eyes. 'Not dead, no… naked.'

'Naked?' There was a brief pause. 'How naked?'

'Completely, utterly and entirely naked.' Kate moved away from the wall, making certain she was alone. 'I walked in on Calvin coming out of the shower.'

'As in, the good-looking bloke you're working for?'

'That's the one.'

Beth burst out laughing.

'It's not funny.'

'Are you kidding me? It's hilarious. Why did you scream?'

Good question. Why had she screamed?

She walked across the gravel courtyard and focused on the views ahead: rolling fields glittering with frost, the surrounding trees clinging on to their few remaining leaves. The serenity of it was enough to ease the thumping in her chest. 'I didn't know I had. Shock, probably.'

'Good shock, or bad shock? Was he hot?'

The heat in her cheeks intensified, despite the chilly November air. 'No comment, on the grounds that I may incriminate myself.'

'That good, huh?' Beth continued to laugh. 'Oh, well, it's one way to brighten your day. How are you feeling now? Have you recovered?'

'Not in the least. I doubt that he has, either. Poor man.' The recollection of his expression when he'd spotted her standing there made her cringe. 'He looked kind of unhappy about being gawped at.'

'Can't say I blame him. I'd feel the same. But I wouldn't worry, he'll get over it. Men don't have the same hang-ups about their bodies as women do. Not the men I know, anyway. He's probably flattered.'

'I doubt that. He looked mortified.' Kate fanned her face, trying to cool her burning skin. In the distance, a couple of horses galloped across the field, their warm breath visible against the pale sky. 'Anyway, did you call for a reason?'

'Only to check up on you. How's it going? You know, apart from walking in on a hot naked bloke.' She laughed again.

Kate was glad someone found it funny.

'Are you making progress with probate?'

She sighed. 'Not really. It's painstakingly slow, hindered by my poor accountancy skills and inability to make sense of the business finances.'

'Why are you getting involved with the business? Don't they have an accountant?'

'Yes, but he's refusing to do any more work until his bill is paid. The business is in debt, but it's still a viable asset, so it needs to be included in the probate application. Trying to calculate its value is impossible… there're too many variables. It's doing my head in.' Kate watched the horses disappear into the distance. 'I've listed two garage blocks for auction next month, in the hope of freeing up some cash and paying the accountant, but the books need sorting out quicker than that.'

'Why don't you ask Alex to help? My brother's not exactly busy at the moment. He's still trying to "find himself". Whatever that means. He could do with something to focus on. He must've picked up some useful knowledge before quitting his accountancy degree.'

Whether her cousin Alex would prove a help or a hindrance, she didn't know. He was laid-back to the point of horizontal and partial to smoking the occasional joint. Inviting his input might create another problem she didn't need. Still, he knew more than she did about balancing books, so maybe it was worth the risk. 'I have no money to pay him.'

'I wouldn't worry about that — it's not like he's earning anything lying around Mum's place, is it? It'll do him good to get off his backside and make himself useful. Besides, Mum's eager for some space so she can entertain her latest boy-toy.'

'Don't you mean toy-boy?'

'Not on this occasion. But the less said about that, the better. Anyway, she'll be glad to get rid of Alex for a bit, he's cramping her style. Shall I talk to him? No harm in asking.'

Kate wondered if she should check with Calvin first, but that would involve talking to the man – something she was keen to avoid doing for the next decade. 'Go on then, but tell him I can't pay him until after probate's been granted.'

'Leave it with me. By the way, I have news. Megan and Zac are expecting a baby.'

'A baby?' Kate felt the instant prick of tears sting her eyes. 'Megan's pregnant?'

'It's due in April. How exciting is that?'

'Super exciting.' Kate hoped the wobble in her voice wouldn't betray her.

It was strange how a piece of news could evoke both instant joy and crippling pain. She was delighted for her cousin – of course she was – it was what both Megan and Zac wanted, and she was over the moon for them. But at the same time a slicing pain sneaked between her ribs. She'd wanted children so badly. A family had been what her and Tristan had both wanted… or so she'd thought.

In the early days, Tristan had reasoned that they needed to get settled first and set up home. Then he'd wanted to focus on his business, and ensure they had a stable and regular income. Then he claimed to be concerned about raising a baby in a high-rise in Clapham. One excuse after another; reasons why they shouldn't start trying and should wait a while longer – reasons that flew out the window when she'd discovered he'd impregnated their next-door neighbour.

Kate was thirty-two years old and painfully single. It seemed like her dream of having a family of her own was slipping away faster than she'd run from Calvin Johnson's bedroom. It was hard not to feel aggrieved.

'They're beyond thrilled,' Beth said, oblivious to her cousin's anguish. 'I'm going to be an aunty.'

'That's great news, Beth. I'm so pleased for you.' Kate managed to force the words past the tightness in her throat. 'Send my congratulations, if you speak to them.'

'I will… hang on a sec…' Beth disappeared for a few moments. 'Sorry, got to go. Dad needs to talk to me about a client. He says hi, by the way, and sends his love. I'll call you later, after I've spoken to Alex. Oh… and Kate? Next time you walk in on Calvin Johnson naked, try not to scream, okay? It's not good for a man's ego.'

'Funny.'

Beth ended the call, still laughing.

Lost in thought, Kate almost jumped out of her skin when the kitchen door slammed behind her. She turned to see the infamous Rowan Blakely walking towards her. At least he wasn't dressed as the Scarlet Pimpernel this time. Although, he still made quite the impact – his tweed suit contrasted with his woollen turquoise waistcoat, whose colour matched the silk scarf around his neck, and he carried a fancy walking cane.

'Good day, young lady. And how are we today? Feeling on top form, I hope. I'm Rowan Blakely.' He extended his hand. 'We've yet to be formally introduced.'

'Kate Lawrence.' She shook his gloved hand. 'Pleased to meet you.'

'Apologies for the other night when, I believe, I gave you quite the fright. Our esteemed new owner told me off for going off the rails, but one does like to shake things up a bit at my age. The time for playing it safe has long gone. It's excitement and adventure from now on.'

Kate couldn't help smiling. Maybe she should follow Rowan's philosophy, instead of her own mournful musings. 'It's fine, I just wasn't expecting to see a face at the window. I had no idea you were even in the car.'

He laughed. 'I'd been on one of my jaunts. One does likes to dress the part when re-enacting a dramatic scenario. Are you a believer?'

She frowned. 'As in religion?'

'Goodness, no. The paranormal. Ghosts?'

'Oh, right. Very much a non-believer.'

He removed a handkerchief from his top pocket. 'Shame, you have quite the aura.'

'I do?'

He looked her up and down. 'Are you sure you've never crossed over to the other side?'

'Quite sure.'

'You'll have to come along to one of my meetings at The Black Horse Inn. You know what they say: forewarned is fore-armed. It's better you know what to expect than be caught unaware. Most people visit Pluckley without stirring the spirits, but I'm guessing that's not the case with you.' He pinned her with a serious look. 'Tell me about the screaming.'

Oh, heavens, had he heard her scream when she'd walked in on Calvin?

'The night you arrived in Pluckley. You heard something, didn't you? Emanating from the woods?'

Phew, he hadn't heard her. And then the penny dropped. Hang on, how did he know about that? 'It was just the wind playing tricks.'

'Oh…? You didn't hear a piercing scream, followed by a cacophony of bird wings flapping?' Using his hand, he mimicked a bird flying off.

'Of… of course not,' she lied, finding it hard to swallow.

'Shame, I felt a kindred spirit had arrived. Especially when I saw you staring into the woods, a look of panic on your face, as though you'd seen him.'

'Who?'

'The Highwayman.'

Kate raised an eyebrow. 'The Highwayman?'

'At last, I thought, someone who can confirm his existence. Do you know the legend?'

'Er… no, I don't.'

'Then let me enlighten you.'

Kate wasn't sure she had much choice.

Rowan held his cane aloft. 'The Highwayman legend tells of a roguish womaniser who met his gruesome end whilst robbing a member of the local gentry on the road past Fright Corner. The unsuspecting victim turned out to be an accomplished swordsman and a fight ensued.'

Kate checked her surroundings, fearing Rowan's loud voice might invite onlookers. Or at least, scare off the cows in the neighbouring field.

'The clash of battling swords can still be heard at the fatal scene where the Highwayman's life came to a sudden end.' He lunged forwards, making her step backwards.

She did not want to be stabbed, thank you very much.

'So, too, can the agonising scream arising from his lips as his assailant's blade pierced his body, pinning it to the trunk of an old hollow tree and sending the birds flapping manically into the night sky.'

She couldn't fault Rowan's enthusiasm, even if it was a little intense.

He advanced on her, making her back away even further. 'Did you see it?'

'Did I see what?'

'His dark shadowy outline lingering close to where the tree once stood.'

'Can't say that I did.' Kate was now backing away at speed. That was, until Calvin's voice startled her.

'Here you are,' he said behind her, making her jump.

'Jesus,' she said, swinging around to face him, almost relieved that she had a valid excuse for her flustered state. 'What is it with you people? You gave me such a fright.' She rubbed her chest, trying to ease her racing heartbeat. 'You're as bad as him.' She nodded to where a grinning Rowan was taking a deep bow, congratulating himself on his performance.

'Sorry, I didn't mean to sneak up on you,' Calvin said, with a half-hearted shrug. 'It's not nice when someone catches you unawares, is it?' His head tilted to one side and she wasn't sure whether the slight edge in his voice had a hint of amusement or accusation.

Either way, it shamed her into a blush. 'I'm really sorry about that. I had no idea it was your room.'

'Maybe knock next time?'

Next time? There wasn't going to be a next time. She'd be steering well clear of his room in future.

Calvin turned to Rowan. 'Have you been telling scary stories again?'

'Nothing that isn't true, dear boy.' Rowan tipped his hat.

Calvin rolled his eyes. 'Try not to scare her too much, I need her.'

'So I've heard,' Rowan said with an exaggerated wink. 'Esme's been filling me in.'

'I'll bet she has.' Shaking his head, Calvin turned to Kate. He was fully dressed now, looking warm and cosy in his hooded jacket and dark jeans. His hair was tied up, but it was still damp from the shower. It seemed to have expanded in size, looking all soft and bouncy, and for a fleeting moment she wondered what it would be like to touch. 'I'm heading into Ashford to pick up supplies. Will you be okay for a while without me?'

Embarrassed at where her thoughts had been headed, she shook away the image, and nodded. 'Sure, no problem. I just came out here for some air... you know, after I... well, after I couldn't get a phone signal inside.'

'So you said.' If she wasn't mistaken, his cheeks were slightly flushed. She wasn't the only one embarrassed. 'See you later, then.' He hesitated, before walking off.

'Right. Yes, bye.' She could relax... and then she remembered her conversation with Beth. 'Calvin!' She ran after him. 'Would it be okay if my cousin came to stay for a while? His accountancy skills are better than mine and I could do with the help. I'll pay him out of my commission, obviously. I don't expect you to cover his costs, but it would definitely speed things up. Would that be okay?'

'Sure, whatever you need. Let me know when he's due to arrive and I'll make up a room for him.'

'Thanks… See you later, then.' She backed away, almost tripping over a raised tree root. What was it with this place? 'I'd better get back to work. Nice to meet you, Rowan.'

Rowan gave a deep bow. 'My pleasure entirely, dear lady.' His gaze drifted from her to Calvin. 'Your arrival has certainly shaken things up. I predict fun times ahead.' He threw back his head and laughed. 'How thrilling.'

Not quite the word she'd use. 'Disturbing' would be a better description.

Kate scurried inside – her face still hot and her heart racing – hoping she wasn't about to have another meltdown… and wondering what exactly had happened that night in Screaming Woods. Was she really a magnet for all things spectral?

She bloody-well hoped not.

That was the last thing she needed.

Chapter Eight

Thursday nights used to be mates' nights. Fridays and Saturdays were off limits, as he usually had a match the next day and was under strict instructions to eat well, abstain from partying and be in bed at a reasonable hour. He valued his career too much to bend the rules, so he'd obediently stuck to the schedule, much to Ainsley's frustration; she'd enjoyed nothing more than a night clubbing in Leeds at the weekend. But Thursday nights were reserved for his mates, having a curry or going to a bar. He liked a beer as much as the next guy.

Since moving to Pluckley, his Thursday nights were like every other night, spent in the company of disillusioned staff and eccentric octogenarians. How his life had changed.

'Here he is,' Esme announced, as he entered the lounge. 'Did you have any luck?'

'All done,' he said, handing her the glasses, which she immediately placed on the side table, not wanting to be seen wearing them unless she absolutely had to.

'You're an angel,' she said, patting his hand. Granny Esme was looking very stylish, in a black velvet jacket over a long grey dress – her dark red lipstick the only splash of colour to her sophisticated outfit.

'They should be okay now. A screw had come loose.'

'Story of my life,' Rowan said, sipping his brandy. 'I've had a screw loose since the day my mother dropped me on my head.'

'Well, that explains a lot,' Geraldine said, making the rest of them laugh.

Rowan stroked his wine-coloured cravat. 'It's made me who I am, darling. Unique.'

'That's one word for it.' Geraldine leant down and stroked Suki, who was curled up asleep on the rug by her feet. '"Bonkers" would be another.'

'And here I was, thinking you enjoyed my *ubiquitous* outlook on life.' Rowan waved his hand, almost knocking over a candle that was balanced on the coffee table.

Esme frowned. 'Is that the right word?'

Calvin had no idea. Judging by the looks on everyone else's faces, they didn't either.

He had to admit they looked a cosy group: sitting around the lounge, filling the worn leather sofas, and looking content as they sipped their drinks and enjoyed the open fire.

Lucky Larry was playing the grand piano – something he did every evening after dinner, providing a mellow backdrop to their gathering and showcasing his talent as a former blues musician. Perhaps this was what his granny had been missing back in Leeds. Like-minded people who had reached their twilight years, but who still had an appetite for good wine and good company, and weren't above getting up to no good. He could imagine them causing havoc in their younger days, breaking rules and spicing up any gathering.

He realised they were all looking at him. 'What have I done?'

'It's what you haven't done,' Geraldine said, hauling herself up from the sofa.

'Did I miss something on the list?' He'd been working flat out all day, trying to make himself useful and placate the staff. He had run errands, which included taking Larry to his audiology appointment... something he would've done anyway, even without Hanna's threat to quit. While he wasn't entirely convinced she'd actually leave, he didn't want to put that theory to the test. They couldn't survive without Hanna, which was probably the reason why she'd upped the ante by making threats. Do something, or she was off.

She was right, though: things weren't good, which was why he was busting a gut, trying to fit in as many chores as possible. Chores he'd never done before, like cleaning dentures, ironing bedsheets, bagging up clinical waste and learning how to use a hoist.

'What do you need, Geraldine? Only, I'm heading off to the station to collect Kate's cousin. I can deal with it if it's a quick one.'

'It is,' she said, sliding her arm around his waist. 'One dance will do me wonders. Play us something smoochy, Larry.'

Calvin looked down in horror, as Geraldine rested her head on his chest and began swaying. Both arms were around him, preventing an escape. 'I'm not the best person to dance with,' he said, as he was dragged into a slow shuffle.

'Nonsense,' Esme said, smiling. 'You were on the dance floor all night at your sister's wedding.'

That was different. Partly because he'd been drinking all day, but mostly because everyone danced at weddings. It wasn't the same as slow-dancing with a handsy older woman, while being watched by his smirking granny and a delighted-looking Rowan, who was humming along to the music. 'They don't make music like the good old days,' he said, tapping his foot to the rhythm.

'Oh, I don't know. I quite like a bit of Stormzy myself.' Esme caught Calvin's eye. 'I've been known to vossi bop.'

Smiling, Calvin remembered his sister's wedding reception; it was a sight he'd never forget.

'Maybe not so good to foxtrot to, though,' Esme said, reaching for her wine.

'Your great-uncle and I used to dance like this,' Geraldine said, tightening her grip. 'He was a spectacular dancer. Knew all the right moves.' She tilted her head up. 'I do miss him, you know.' Tears pooled in her eyes and Calvin felt mean for resenting dancing with her. He resigned himself to finishing the dance, praying her hands would stay on his back and not wander any lower.

When the song ended, he freed himself from Geraldine's clasp and made his excuses to leave. 'I'd better check on Kate,' he said, heading for the door. 'Enjoy your evening, everyone.'

'Who am I going to dance with now?' Geraldine called after him.

'I'll dance with you, Geraldine.' Rowan got up and offered her his hand. 'Shall we?'

Calvin left them to their dancing and headed for the library.

It was unsurprising to find Kate still working at gone nine p.m. The woman was relentless. She rarely took a break, and even when she did, it was only because Esme or Geraldine insisted that she eat something. He probably should do more to ensure her wellbeing, but he was so busy that he barely had time to speak to her... which was just an excuse.

Until Tuesday morning, he'd had no problem chatting to her. It was true he found her attractive, but there hadn't been any awkwardness between them. He'd helped her with logging the estate assets and answered any questions she had. But from the moment she'd walked in on him getting out of the shower, he'd avoided her. He didn't know why – he guessed he was just embarrassed.

He'd felt exposed and vulnerable, standing there naked, which wasn't logical. As a footballer, getting his kit off in front of people was part of everyday life. But somehow this was different: she wasn't a teammate or a disinterested physio carrying out medical checks – she was a smart, professional, attractive woman who was working for him. So when she'd flushed bright red, gawped at him and stumbled from the room like he had two heads, his self-esteem had taken another blow. But he couldn't avoid her forever.

As he entered the library, for a moment he couldn't work out where she was... until she yelped. He looked up to find her swinging from one of the bookcase doors. 'Jesus! Don't let go,' he said, grabbing the stepladders and rolling them under her.

'Oh, great advice,' she yelled down, her voice drier than sandpaper. 'I hadn't thought of that. Silly me.'

Okay, so she was mad. It was hardly his fault, was it? He climbed up the ladder and grabbed hold of her legs. 'Why didn't you use the stepladders?'

She growled and twisted her head to make eye contact with him. 'Of course I used the bloody stepladders, I'm not an idiot.'

He was eye level with her midriff, looking up at her angry expression. Her cheeks were pink and she was breathing heavily. 'Then how come they weren't underneath you?'

'Oh, I don't know, maybe because the bloody things moved.'

'Moved?'

'Yes, moved. One moment they were under me, the next they'd shifted out of reach.'

He raised an eyebrow. 'Maybe you knocked them?'

'Or maybe they have a mind of their own. Like the window that keeps banging open, or the picture on the wall that keeps winking at me.'

Tiredness was affecting her mental state, clearly. 'Winking at you?'

'Yes, you know...' She blinked at him furiously and he tried not to laugh. 'Like someone is toying with my sanity and deliberately trying to sabotage my efforts to catalogue this bloody estate.'

She nodded at the painting, which remained just as it was: an ancient portrait of a pompous army general, his expression static.

She growled again. 'Typical, he's not going to do it now that there's someone else in the room. That's right,' she yelled at the painting. 'Make me out to be unhinged. Thanks for that.'

'Kate...?' He waited until she looked at him. She was teetering on the verge of a meltdown, and he wasn't sure he could hold on to her if she collapsed. 'How about we climb down and get you on solid ground?'

Her frown didn't let up as she stared at him, her light blue eyes fixed on his, slightly unfocused. 'You think I'm a crazy person, don't you?'

'I think you've been working crazy hours,' he said, trying to be tactful. 'You're tired and stressed, and I'll bet you haven't stopped for a break all day. Your hands are freezing and you're shaking. Nobody can keep going the way you do. It's time you stopped for the night, okay?'

She gave a reluctant nod. 'But the stepladders did move, I'm not making it up.'

'I believe you. Can you hold the ladder?' He took her cold hand and placed it on the top rung. 'That's it, now move your left foot across.' He edged his body away from the ladder, allowing her enough space to squeeze between him and the rungs. 'Let go of your right hand and swing yourself across, okay? I've got you.'

She did as he asked and tentatively manoeuvred herself onto the ladder, which creaked beneath them. Jesus, he hoped it wouldn't collapse under their combined weight.

So much for avoiding any unnecessary interactions. His body was pressed against her back, his arms stretched around her while holding on to the ladder. They couldn't be any more intimate if they tried. If she hadn't been shaking and clearly upset, he would have moved away. As it was, he focused on holding the ladder steady, ignoring the sensation of her bum pressing into his midriff. 'Are you secure?'

'I'm fine.' She didn't sound it.

'You're not going to fall, okay? I'm right here.'

When she nodded, her hair tickled his nose, making him sneeze. 'Bless you.'

'Thank you.' And he'd thought his life couldn't get any more surreal. 'I'm heading down, okay?'

Each step he took, she did the same, which meant that her bum continued to bump against him as they descended. When they eventually reached the floor, he stepped away. There was only so much torment his body could take.

There hadn't been anyone since Ainsley, and he'd be lying if he said he didn't miss physical intimacy. He could feel his skin beginning to warm and grow more sensitive, and the overwhelming urge to reach out and touch her was highly disturbing.

Needing to break the moment, he stepped further away, creating even more space between them. She'd triggered a memory, that was all. The buzz in his blood was a reflex, his body aching to feel close to another human being. It wasn't anything more than a physical craving and the desire to feel something other than grief. He missed Ainsley, that was all. It had nothing to do with Kate.

When Kate reached the bottom, she turned to him. 'Thanks for helping me.'

'That's okay. How do you feel?'

'Foolish,' she said, rubbing her chest. Her breathing was shallow and she grimaced every time she took a breath. 'But I swear I'm not lying about the ladders. They moved.' She looked upset and confused, and he felt rotten for her.

He made a quick decision. 'I'm heading into the village to pick up Alex from the station, do you want to come with me? It might do you good to get out of here for a while. I'm sure you're keen to see your cousin.'

Her confusion deepened. 'Is it that time already? I had no idea.'

'Like I said, you've been working too hard. Do you need anything before we go? A hot drink? Something to eat?'

She hesitated, as if tempted, but shook her head. 'I'm not up to dealing with Geraldine tonight. I'll make myself something later when she's gone home. Sorry if that sounds mean, but she can be a bit full on at times.'

'Tell me about it. I've just been made to slow-dance with her, while Rowan, Larry and my granny looked on.'

Kate smiled for the first time that evening and some of the tension seemed to leave her. 'I guess I should be grateful she just wants to feed me.'

'You're getting off lightly,' he said, heading over to the door, listening to ensure the others were still in the lounge and wouldn't catch them escaping. 'We're safe. Come on.'

He held the door for her as she tiptoed past and they scurried across the reception to the front door, relieved to have made it outside without being cornered.

The cold hit him as they headed for his car and he regretted not stopping to pick up his jacket. Kate was shivering, too, wrapping her long cardigan around her as she jogged towards his car.

The weather had definitely turned colder. Walking Suki each morning was a test of his character – the dog's, too. She'd glare up at him in indignation at being made to venture out in the cold. Tough, they both needed the exercise.

Turning up the heater, he switched on the heated seats and pulled away from the care home, heading for the village.

Kate leant against the headrest, her breathing yet to settle.

'People have started putting up their Christmas lights,' he said, hoping to distract her. 'Over there, see?' He nodded to where a row of houses were lit up by flashing lights, each one seeming to outdo its neighbour with their displays.

Kate rolled her head to look. 'I bet they didn't buy their decorations from the pound shop.'

'This area certainly isn't short of money,' he said, glancing over. 'What were Christmases like when you were young?'

She shrugged. 'A bit of a mixed bag, really.' She fell silent, and for a moment, he didn't think she was going to elaborate, but then she said, 'Mum and I used to go to my aunt and uncle's house in Godalming for Christmas. They lived in this big posh place, with fancy white furnishings and seven bedrooms, even though there were only five of them.' Her face creased into a frown as she looked over at him. 'Is my bum getting warm?'

He nodded. 'Heated seats.'

She let out a whistle. 'Crikey, my last car didn't even have a working fan.' She shifted position. 'I was worried I'd wet myself.'

He laughed. 'If you have, let me know and I'll increase the settings. You'll dry out in no time.'

'Wow, how the other half live.' She was smiling, so he figured she was teasing.

They drove past St Nicholas's church, with its graveyard illuminated by the neighbouring festive lights. 'You were telling me about Christmases at your aunt and uncle's house?'

'Oh, right, yes.' She turned away and looked out of the window. 'Well, they used to have caterers in to cook Christmas dinner, and the decorations were all handcrafted, from this fancy posh boutique in Godalming. Aunty Connie would pick a different colour scheme each year and spend a fortune creating a theme. We'd get taken to the carols at the Royal Albert Hall, ice-skating in Hyde Park, and there'd always be a sack of presents waiting for me on Christmas morning.'

He glanced over. 'Sounds idyllic.'

'You'd think,' she said, with a deep sigh.

'It wasn't?'

'I always felt sorry for my mum. She never said anything, and she acted as though she was delighted I was getting spoilt so much, but I could tell it hurt her.'

'How come?'

'Because she couldn't offer me the same.' Another pause, as if she was debating how much to say. 'We didn't have much money when I was growing up. It was just the two of us, and Mum had to work several jobs to pay the rent. She couldn't take time off during school holidays to look after me, so I was sent to stay with my cousins. I had a great time, don't get me wrong – I love my extended family, but I always missed my mum. I knew she hated not being able to make a better life for us. So… you know… things like Christmas were always bittersweet.'

He was shocked by how similar their upbringings had been. His family hadn't had any money, either. If it hadn't been for his granny and Uncle Bert, they wouldn't have had regular heating, let alone Christmas presents. 'Your dad wasn't around?'

She paused before answering. 'My dad died when I was a baby.'

'I'm sorry, Kate. That's grim.' He hadn't had a dad either, although his wasn't dead, just absent. 'Was it an accident?' He turned into the parking bay outside the pub.

'No, not an accident,' she said, straining to see out of the window. 'Why have we stopped? This isn't the train station.'

'You need feeding.' He opened the driver's door when it became clear that nothing more was forthcoming about her dad.

Her eyes grew wide. 'You don't need—'

'I know,' he cut her off. 'But I haven't eaten either and I'm starving. Even if you don't need food, I do.'

'Fine,' she said, unclipping her seat belt. 'Do we have time before Alex's train arrives?'

He checked his watch. 'We've got half an hour. I'll ask them to serve us quickly.'

They exited the car and headed up the pub steps.

The Black Horse Inn was a sombre building, with shuttered windows and an array of blackened horseshoes framing the doorway. As they reached the entrance, the large pub sign rattled loudly.

Kate glanced up, her eyes narrowing at the fierce-looking black beast gazing down at her. 'What is it with this place and their creaky signs? Hasn't anyone ever heard of WD-40?'

Smiling, he opened the door. 'I told you, it adds to the ambience. The tourists love it.'

'I'll be they do.' The door creaked as it swung open and Kate paused to look at him. 'I doubt the props department working on a film would go to this much trouble to recreate a haunted set.' She turned to walk off, but then looked back at him. 'Are you sure you haven't adopted some of these gimmicks back at the care home? Moving ladders? An unreliable fireplace? Creaky windows?'

He grinned at her. 'Why would we do that?'

94

'Oh, I don't know. Give the new person a hard time. Keep her on her toes. Freak her out, and then sit back and laugh as she unravels.'

'That would be like shooting myself in the foot. I need you, remember?'

'Right. I keep forgetting.' She pointed to an empty table by the fireplace. 'Over there?'

'Head over and I'll order at the bar. They do a great burger. Do you eat red meat?'

'Occasionally.' She gave a quick shrug. 'Burger sounds good. A beer, too, please. Whatever lager they have on tap.'

'Coming up.'

The inside of the pub was warm and homely. A Christmas tree filled one corner, its coloured lights pulsating in time with the festive music playing softly in the background.

He watched as Kate shrugged off her cardigan and threw it over the back of a chair. Removing the elastic band from her hair, she let it fall loose onto her shoulders and ran her hands through it, as though she was trying to force her body to relax. The bright lick of flames from the fireplace bathed her in a soft glow and he was so mesmerised for a moment that he almost didn't hear the barman asking him what he wanted.

Having ordered their food, he carried the drinks over to Kate. 'Ten minutes for the burgers.' He placed a beer in front of her. 'How are you feeling?'

'You mean, have I stopped imagining the care home is possessed by poltergeists?'

He sat down and observed her cautiously. 'Is that what you believe is happening?'

She gave him a sarcastic look. 'Credit me with some sanity. I have no idea what's wrong with the place, but I don't for one moment think it's haunted.'

He let out a breath. 'Thank goodness for that. You had me worried there.'

'Why, were you concerned I might be emotionally unstable?' She took a long sip of beer. 'Sadly, that ship's already sailed, as you know only too well… Nice beer, cheers.' She lifted her glass.

'Cheers.' He clinked glasses with her. 'Is being here in Kent making it worse?'

She seemed to mull over the question. 'Strangely, no… although I've no idea why. It's not exactly a restful place, or an easy job, but at least it's keeping me occupied. Hopefully, it'll result in me being debt-free soon, so it's worth the effort.' She rested her arms on the table and studied him. 'Can I ask you a question?'

He relaxed back in his chair. 'Fire away.'

'How come you're not playing football at the moment?'

The question caught him off guard and he lowered his eyes, suddenly transfixed by his beer. 'How do you mean?'

'Isn't it the middle of the football season? I was curious as to how come you're not playing.'

It was a fair enough question and he lifted his eyes to meet hers. 'How do you know I was a footballer?'

She gave him a sheepish look. 'I googled you. And before you accuse me of invading your privacy again, I was carrying out due diligence. There's no way I was going to move here and accept a job without checking you out first. If you remember, you just showed up at my door unannounced. I had no idea who you were until I searched your name.'

He took a long slug of beer, needing a hit of alcohol to dull the ache that had crept into his chest.

Thankfully, the waiter arrived with their burgers, and he was given a few moments' respite to compose himself while sauces and cutlery were being sorted out.

He waited until the waiter had disappeared, before replying. 'If you googled me, then you would've read about why I'm no longer playing football.'

'To be fair, I didn't read much,' she said, placing a napkin across her lap. 'I just saw the main headlines about you playing for Leeds Park United and what a local hero you were. Stuff like that.' She took a bite of burger and her eyelids fluttered closed in appreciation. 'Oh, that's good,' she said, washing it down with a mouthful of beer. 'Your girlfriend is very beautiful, by the way.' She ate some more burger, oblivious to the injury her words had caused him.

He picked up his burger, but the tightness in his throat meant that eating wasn't an option, so he placed it back on the plate.

'So having read about your successful career,' she said, swallowing a mouthful of food, 'I was curious as to how you ended up here, dealing with your uncle's estate?'

He rubbed his forehead. 'Wow, you really didn't read much, did you?'

She wiped her mouth with the napkin. 'Did something happen? Are you injured?'

'You could say that.' He took another mouthful of beer, no longer hungry and needing a moment before replying.

The words never got any easier to say, no matter how many times he'd said them. He could change the subject and avoid answering, but what was the point? Why shouldn't she know the truth? Everyone else at the care home did. It wasn't fair to keep her in the dark.

'My girlfriend is now my ex-girlfriend, and I'm not playing football anymore, because I'm no longer allowed to. I'm considered a liability.'

She frowned at him. 'Why on earth would you be a liability?' And then she lifted her hand. 'Sorry, you don't have to tell me, it's none of my business. Forget I said anything. Let's enjoy our food.'

Lowering her gaze, she returned to eating her burger, and he was left debating whether or not to continue. Tempting as it was to let it go, he didn't want things to be any more awkward between them than they already were. He might as well tell her the full story.

Besides, she'd probably only google him again, and he'd rather she heard it from him than read the sensationalist spin the tabloids had put on it. According to some news reports, he was already as good as dead. 'It's okay, you weren't to know,' he said, pushing his plate away, his appetite now completely gone. 'I have a heart condition. It's called hypertrophic cardiomyopathy. HCM for short. It means my heart could suddenly stop at any moment, triggered by extreme exercise.'

She stopped eating and looked at him, eyes wide. 'Well, that's a bit shit, isn't it?'

He had to smile at that. 'It is a bit shit, yes.'

She picked up the napkin and wiped her hands. 'And there's nothing they can do to stop that happening?'

'I have a device fitted in my chest that'll restart my heart if it stops, but it's not enough to convince the Football Association to insure me.'

Her face dropped. 'So that's it? Game over?'

'Game over.'

She sat back in her chair. 'When did this happen?'

'June this year. This is the first season I'm not playing football since I was five years old. My life has only ever been about football. And now, nothing. Gone.'

A beat passed before she spoke, as if she was trying to figure out what to say. What could she say? There were no words of consolation that would ease the sorrow he felt. It was a permanent wound, one he feared he might never recover from.

She reached across and touched his hand. Her noticed that her hand was no longer cold. 'I'm so sorry, Calvin. That's... heartbreaking.' And then she flinched and withdrew her hand. 'Sorry, that's a really poor choice of word.'

He smiled. 'It's okay. It's better than telling me "it's only a game" and I'll get over it.' He nodded at her burger. 'Eat up or it'll go cold. And can you please stop looking at me like that?'

'Like what?'

'Like you feel sorry for me.'

'Well, I do.' She pushed her plate away, as if making a point.

'It's not like anyone died. I had a good career, a good income, and I got to experience some amazing things. I should feel grateful. Especially when I look at Priya and Deshad in the care home. My situation is nothing compared to theirs.'

'That doesn't mean you're not entitled to feel aggrieved. You've suffered a horrible loss. The thing you love most in the world has been taken away from you. Don't underestimate the impact of that.' Her expression softened. 'Did you know you had a heart condition?'

He shook his head. 'No idea. It came out of the blue.'

'Then you're also dealing with the shock of your diagnosis and the loss of your health. That alone is traumatic… And your girlfriend? Did that happen at the same time?'

He nodded.

She puffed out her cheeks. 'Then, frankly, it's a wonder you're still functioning. Most people would've struggled to get out of bed each day, let alone deal with their family's estate and help others. That's way beyond what most of us could do, even without dealing with what you're going through.' Her knee touched his under the table, which was oddly comforting. 'I know a little about loss and grief, and you've suffered three blows in short succession. That's going to knock the stuffing out of anyone, and it's not like you've had time to process it. I imagine the pain is still very raw and disabling.'

She was right about that. He could feel the emotion building within him even now, but he was not about to start crying in front of Kate Lawrence. He had some pride.

'Is anyone helping you? Like a counsellor, or something?'

He shook his head. 'I don't need counselling, I just need to work out what the hell I'm going to do with my life.'

'Right. And managing the care home isn't it?'

'Christ, no.' He checked his watch, eager to escape the conversation. 'We'd better head off. Alex's train will be arriving… You haven't finished your burger.'

'I've had enough, thanks. It was delicious. You were right, I did need feeding. I'm feeling a lot better.'

'Glad it helped.' He stood up, eager for some fresh air. 'I'll settle the bill.'

'But you haven't touched yours. Shall we ask for a doggy bag?'

'I'm not as hungry as I thought.'

'That's my fault – I shouldn't have been so nosey.' She pulled on her cardigan.

'It's fine, really. It's better you know.'

She caught his arm when he went to walk away. 'I really am sorry, Calvin. Let me know if I can help in any way.'

He forced himself to adopt a neutral expression. 'You're already helping. That's why I hired you. I can't deal with the estate on my own, and the sooner I get everything resolved, the sooner I can go home to Leeds and rebuild my life.'

'Right. Understood.' She let go of his arm. 'I'll do everything I can to make that happen.'

'Thanks.' Although, right at that moment, heading home no longer felt like the quick fix he'd hoped it would be.

The weight in his stomach seemed to be getting worse, not better.

Chapter Nine

Monday, 6th December

Kate stared at the spreadsheet on her laptop, trying to absorb the enormity of the information she'd collated. It was definitely a case of two steps forwards, one step back. On a positive note, she was making good headway in listing the estate's assets. On the negative side, she'd spent the last three days buried deep in paperwork, which had revealed a number of issues – mainly a significant gap between the care home's income and the care home's expenditure.

Still, it wasn't all bad. She'd heard back from the Land Registry about the leasehold properties in London, and thanks to Alex's help, she had a better understanding of the care home's overall finances. Baby steps, and all that.

The library door opened and a flustered-looking Alex appeared. 'Well, that was fun,' he said, flopping onto the window seat, his long skinny frame too big for the narrow space.

Kate swivelled the office chair, so she was facing him. 'It didn't go well?'

'It couldn't have gone worse,' he said, shuffling into a sitting position. 'That woman is completely unreasonable. Not to mention illogical. And… really, really annoying.'

'I take it you're referring to Hanna, not Natalie?'

'Natalie was fine. She understood exactly where I was coming from. But Hanna reacted as though I was accusing her of grand larceny. All I said was that if you added up the rent costs for staying in a place like this, including utilities, food and

Council Tax, then it came to more than her monthly salary. So even though she isn't getting paid, she is getting a good deal by staying here rent-free.'

'She didn't see it that way?'

Alex pointed to his forehead. 'She threw a bedpan at me.'

Kate flinched.

'I ducked... but it was a close call. I thought if I explained that she wasn't being ripped off, she might calm down and see reason. Like Natalie, who totally got it. She said she was grateful Calvin was letting her stay and understood why he couldn't pay her at the moment. But not Hanna – she accused me of being a money-grabbing accountant, who dresses like a scarecrow and needs a haircut. Rude.'

Kate felt for her cousin. Alex had never been blessed with an abundance of confidence, and she couldn't imagine that a feisty woman like Hanna laying into him would help.

Alex had dropped out of university after the first year, claiming that accountancy wasn't for him. His family had a different take on things. They felt his unfocused attitude, regular drug use and heavy drinking were probably bigger factors behind his struggle with his course, rather than a lack of ability to cope with fiscal percentages.

What followed were a tricky few years, when Alex spiralled into depression and addiction, and his parents became more frustrated by his lack of drive and ambition. It didn't help that his sisters were hugely successful in their careers. In fact, the more successful they became, the more Alex seemed to disappear into his shell... until two years ago, when something happened at Megan's wedding that seemed to ignite a change.

To this day, no one knew exactly what happened that weekend. Maybe it was watching his mother recover from an acrimonious divorce to become a successful personal trainer. Or perhaps it was watching Megan and Zac tie the knot in search of a 'happy ever after'. Or maybe Beth was right, and it was something do to with her partner, Matt, intervening and giving

Alex a good talking-to. Whatever the reason, Alex came off the weed, stopped drinking, joined AA and enrolled in college to finish his accountancy course. And no one had been more shocked or surprised than his family.

Consequently, Alex was a changed man. Well, sort of. Despite being thirty-two, he still looked like a floppy-haired teenager, whose clothes never quite fitted his lithe frame, but at least now he was sober, and making an effort to turn things around. Kate just hoped that dealing with the estate accounts wouldn't dent his fragile self-esteem.

'I need some air,' he said, getting up from the window seat. 'I'll walk into the village.' He grabbed his padded parka from the coat stand. 'I won't be long.'

Kate held her breath, praying he wasn't heading for The Black Horse Inn to drown his sorrows. She couldn't bear to be the cause of a relapse.

'I'll visit the butcher's while I'm there and see if I can persuade the owner to extend the care home's credit. He might be more amicable if I ask in person.'

Kate inwardly sighed. 'Good plan. Hope it works.'

'Me too.' Alex headed out, his head hanging low, his shoulders slumped. Working at The Rose Court Care Home was testing all their resolves, it seemed.

Kate headed over to the window and watched him disappear down the driveway.

Had she done the right thing asking Alex for help? She hoped so. He was bound to encounter people like Hanna in the workplace, so he'd need to get used to handling them at some point. Was that enough justification? She wasn't sure.

As she headed back to the desk, she became aware of piano music resonating from the lounge next door. She recognised the song, 'Mack the Knife', played in a slow jazz style, with a flurry of improvised runs overlapping the melody.

Intrigued, she headed next door.

A man she hadn't met before was seated at the piano. He looked distinguished, probably in his late seventies, with curly

Afro hair speckled with grey. He sported a neatly trimmed beard and wore a dark blazer over an open-neck shirt, and he gently swayed as his fingers caressed the piano keys.

Hoping not to startle him, she crept closer and leant against the piano, but when he stopped playing, she stepped away, mortified. 'I'm so sorry, I didn't mean to interrupt.'

'You didn't,' he said, smiling. 'You must be Kate?'

'And I'm guessing you're... Lucky Larry?' He was the only resident she'd yet to meet. 'You play beautifully. Your technique is flawless.'

'I've had lots of practice, been playing for over sixty years. Do you play?'

'Not to your standard.'

'Sit beside me.' He shifted position to make room for her. 'Know any duets?'

'Not really.' She sat down beside him. 'I can read music, but I'm not very good at improvising. Not like you.' She watched him resume playing, fascinated by his dexterity and lightness of touch. He played a few chords, his left hand adding a few runs over the top that created a bluesy seductive sound. 'Where did you learn to play like that?'

'My mother was a classical pianist. We didn't have a lot growing up in New Orleans, but we did have a piano. She taught all six of us to play. Said it was our ticket out of there.'

'And was it?'

He turned to smile at her. 'Ever heard of Count Basie?'

'Of course.'

'I was playing in his orchestra by the age of fifteen.'

'Wow. Seriously?' No wonder he was so good.

'I went on to play for many of the Motown artists during the Sixties. Made quite a name for myself as a session musician.'

'That's incredible.' She watched him play, mesmerised by his technique. 'How did you end up in the UK?'

'A woman.'

Kate tutted. 'Ah, the downfall of many a man.'

He laughed. 'Not in this instance. Francie was the best thing that ever happened to me.' He gave her a wink. 'We moved to her home town of Manchester after we married and I became involved in the Northern Soul scene. You're too young to remember that era, but it was an exciting time.'

'I love Northern Soul.'

'You do? Well, what d'ya know.'

'They had regular Northern Soul nights at the student uni bar. I always wanted to join in with the band, but I never did.'

'Why not?'

She shrugged. 'Lack of confidence. Plus, my boyfriend at the time didn't want me making a fool of myself.'

'Sounds like a jerk.'

'Oh, he was. Shame I didn't realise that before I married him.'

Larry laughed. 'I hope you've divorced him.'

'Of course.' Although, not before he'd almost bankrupted her. 'Do you still play in bands now?'

He shook his head. 'Not since my wife died and I was diagnosed with macular degeneration. I don't see so good these days.'

'I'm sorry. It doesn't seem to have affected your playing.'

'I can still mess around with a few tunes.' He lifted his hands from the keys. 'Your turn.'

Kate shifted away. 'Oh, I couldn't. I'm not in your league.'

'Music isn't a competition, it's about expressing yourself. Show me who you are.' He nodded for her to play something.

Who she was? Well, that was a darned good question. Sadly, she had no idea these days – she was still figuring that one out. But despite her reservations, she found herself tempted. It had been weeks since she'd last played and she missed having a creative outlet for her anxiety.

And besides, there was no one else in the room. It was just her and Lucky Larry, an ally if ever there was one.

Tentatively, she rested her hands on the keys and took a deep breath. He'd asked her to show him who she was, so she began playing the opening bars of 'Someone You Loved', not expecting him to recognise it, but he surprised her by saying, 'Lewis Capaldi? Nice choice.'

Smiling, her fingers loosened, as she relaxed into the song.

He watched her play. 'You have good technique... Relax your shoulders... Lower your elbows... Nice.' And then he began to sing. A soft hum at first, before finding his place in the song and joining in with the lyrics.

His deep voice calmed her further, and she was able to let go a little and feel her way into the music, becoming bolder, less self-conscious.

She hadn't been aware of Calvin entering the room until she glanced up and saw him standing by the doorway. Crikey, how long had he been standing there? She immediately stopped playing, her hands retracting from the keys as if she'd been electrocuted.

'Don't stop,' he said, coming over. 'That was amazing.'

There was no way she could continue – the moment was gone. 'I should get back to work,' she said, hastily getting up from the piano. 'I have a lot to do.'

'You're allowed a break,' he said, looking concerned. 'Don't stop because you think you have to. I didn't mean to disturb you.'

'You didn't. I was just... you know, messing around.' She could feel her cheeks growing warm. 'Like I said, I should be working. It was lovely to meet you, Larry.'

'The pleasure was all mine.' He gave her an informal salute. 'Anytime you fancy a jam, you let me know. It'll be nice to have a fellow musician to play with.'

'Thanks... but I couldn't... I mean, I'm not good enough. Thanks for the tips. I'd better get back to the library. Bye!' She almost ran from the room, her relaxed state blown into a flurry of embarrassment.

She hated anyone seeing her play, especially someone like Calvin. Someone who'd been so successful. But then she remembered his life wasn't quite as charmed as she'd first imagined. He'd suffered his fair share of loss recently and her annoyance at being interrupted softened a fraction.

It was ten minutes before Calvin's head appeared around the library door. She wasn't surprised; she knew it would only be a matter of time before he appeared, but at least he'd given her a few moments' respite.

'Okay to come in?' His apprehensive tone indicated he knew she was upset, but he wasn't sure whether it was his fault.

He hadn't done anything wrong. Her own hang-ups were the problem, not his. 'Of course,' she said, forcing a smile.

'You're musical, then?' He was wearing an orange hoodie with a logo she didn't recognise. It was a colour most people couldn't get away with wearing, but against his darker skin tone, it looked great.

'Nothing like Larry,' she said, with a self-conscious shrug. 'He's lived quite the life, hasn't he?'

Calvin came over to the desk. 'Did he tell you he played for Smokey Robinson?'

'Really? I never even made it to the school band.'

Calvin smiled. 'Did you try?'

'Well... no, but that's beside the point.'

His smile expanded, turning into one of those killer-grins that made his dimples pop and her stomach flip. 'I like your Advent calendar,' he said, accidentally knocking over the card from her mum, when he leant against the desk. As he righted it, he spotted the words inside. 'Katiekins? Is that your nickname?'

'It's what my dad used to call me when I was a baby. It kind of stuck. Mum uses it when she's being sentimental.' Her voice caught on the mention of her dad and she had to clear her throat.

'Sweet.' He straightened the card. 'How are you getting on listing the assets?'

'Good, although I've uncovered a bit of a puzzle.' She showed him the entry in the dusty ledger. 'I found this list of wines, some of which are quite rare. The value could be significant, but it doesn't say where the bottles are stored. I've looked in all the obvious places, but I can't find them. Have they been sold, do you know?'

Calvin shook his head. 'They're in the wine cellar.'

'You have a wine cellar? Where? I couldn't find it.'

'It's hidden,' he said, moving away from the desk. 'Come here, I'll show you.'

Intrigued, she followed him.

'I suppose I should start thinking about what we're going to do here at Christmas,' he said, stopping in front of one of the bookcases. 'The residents deserve something nice – the staff, too.'

He was a thoughtful man, she realised, as well as kind, and she was suddenly curious to know more about him. 'What were Christmases like when you were young?' she said, figuring she'd spilled the beans about her upbringing, so it seemed only fair to redress the balance.

'Nothing fancy,' he said, staring at the bookcase. 'We didn't have expensive presents or go on trips to Lapland like some of the kids at school, but we always had a good time. Mum and Granny Esme would be in the kitchen making dinner, and Uncle Bert would make up silly games.'

She watched him counting books. 'Er... what are you doing?'

'Looking for... Ah, here it is.' He removed a battered book and reached behind it to pull a lever. There was a dull clunking sound, followed by a creak. 'The wine cellar's behind here,' he said, tugging open the bookcase to reveal a staircase.

Kate's eyes grew wide. 'A secret passage?'

Calvin cocked an eyebrow. 'Want to take a look?'

'God, yes.' But then she spotted the rustic stone walls and spiralling staircase. 'It looks a bit spooky. Is it safe?'

'As long as you watch your step. The lighting isn't great and there's no handrail.' He flicked a light switch just inside the door and entered the stairwell.

'So, what kind of games did you play?' she asked, following him into the dim light, and trying not to focus on how steep the steps were.

'There was one called the post-office game. Uncle Bert would invent fake town names and hide little carboard post-boxes around the house, and we'd be given letters to post. The first person to post all their letters won the game.'

She followed him down the narrow staircase. 'I bet you always won.'

'Nope, never.'

'How come?'

'Because I never cheated,' he said, glancing back. 'My brother and sister used to hide the postboxes once they'd posted their letters, so I couldn't post mine. I found one in the washing machine once.'

She laughed. 'That's mean.'

'I didn't mind. I'm only competitive on the football pitch. Poor Mum would nearly be sent flying, with us running about the house trying to find the boxes. She never minded, though, she liked us to have fun. It wasn't always easy for her.'

The temperature had noticeably dropped. 'How come?'

'I guess my childhood was similar to yours, in a way. Dad wasn't around and Mum had to work several jobs to pay the bills. We spent school holidays being looked after by Granny Esme or staying with Uncle Bert here in Kent.'

She stopped walking. 'Can I lean on you? I can't see my footing very well.'

'Sure.' He patted his shoulder, waiting until she'd placed her hand there before selecting the torch function on his phone and aiming it downwards. 'Better?'

'Much better. Thanks.'

He carried on down.

'Why wasn't your dad around?' she asked, ducking under a low-hanging cobweb.

'He disappeared back to Jamaica when I was eight. We haven't seen him since.'

Kate felt for him; she knew what it was like to lose a dad. 'Didn't he keep in touch?'

'Not really. The occasional birthday or Christmas card. The last birthday card he sent me was addressed to my brother, so he's never going to win dad of the year if he can't remember whose birthday it is.'

'I'm sorry.' She could feel the heat seeping through his hoodie, a contrast to the cold stairwell.

He gave a half-hearted shrug. ''Tis what it is.'

They reached the bottom and she was glad to be on firmer ground. A single bulb lit the space, revealing racks of bottles covered in thick dust.

'He did phone me once, when I signed my first professional contract,' he said, walking over to one of the racks. 'Gave me this speech about how proud he was and could I get him tickets for my debut match. He wanted to fly over and take me out for a fancy dinner to celebrate. I was so excited. My dad was going to be at my first game. *Maybe he'll stay*, I thought, and we could be a family again. But then he asked for money. Said as I was earning big bucks, could I help him out with some cash, since he'd run up a few debts.'

Kate's heart sank. 'And did you?'

'Sure. I sent him ten grand from my first pay packet, bought him a first-class ticket to visit and rented him a place in Leeds so he could stay for a while.'

Kate bit her lip, fearing what was coming next. 'He never showed up, did he?'

Calvin shook his head. 'We never heard from him again.'

Her heart broke for him. 'That's awful.'

'It didn't matter. The rest of my family came to my first game – that's all I cared about.' He rubbed dust away from one of the bottles. 'Do you know anything about wine?'

'Not much,' she admitted, looking at the various vintages. 'My aunt does, though. She's a fan of some posh brand that costs a packet. I've never had the heart to tell her it tastes the same as the cheap stuff from the supermarket.'

He laughed. 'Not a connoisseur, huh?'

'Far from it. You?'

'More of a beer man.' He disappeared behind the central racking. 'You don't have to wine-and-dine your clients as a solicitor?'

'Not in my area of law. There is a lot of drinking involved, but it's usually tea rather than alcohol. People often feel overwhelmed or vulnerable, and client meetings are more about consoling than covering aspects of law. I guess that's why I like it. I get a sense of satisfaction from helping people.'

'I imagine you're very good at it,' he said, reappearing from behind the wine rack.

'Why do you say that?'

'You're very kind,' he said, softly. 'And you take pride in your work. I've never known anyone work so hard. You're relentless.'

'I have an ulterior motive,' she said, trying to lighten the moment – his words were threatening to unravel her.

'I think you'd behave like this even if you didn't.'

She swallowed awkwardly. 'Maybe.'

He seemed to study her for a moment, his expression unreadable in the dim light. 'What's the worst part about your job?'

'Oh, that's easy,' she said, relieved to change topic. She'd never taken compliments well. 'Targets. I hate the pressure of having to bill for so many hours a month. Especially as I'm supposed to include the time spent reassuring my clients. It makes it feel a bit mercenary.'

He frowned. 'I hope you're keeping track of the hours you work here?'

'Of course.' She looked away, knowing her answer lacked conviction.

'I'm serious, Kate. I don't want you short-changing yourself.'

'I know. And I will, I promise.' She was such a liar. There was no way she was going to charge him her full rate; it didn't seem fair, not with the care home being in such a precarious position. As long as she came away with enough to clear the tax debt, that was all that mattered.

'Kate...?' She still hadn't turned to face him. 'Katiekins?'

That got her attention. She turned, both eyebrows raised.

'I thought that'd get your attention. You need to bill for every hour you work here, okay? Don't do me any favours.' He reached out and touched her arm. 'Please?'

She gave an exaggerated eye-roll. 'Fine. I'll bill for every hour.' The intensity in his gaze was unnerving. She returned to admiring the wine. It was safer that way.

He stepped over a wine crate. 'What about your mum? How's she doing these days?'

'Oh, she's okay. She's with a lovely man called Brian, who worships the ground she walks on. She's happy, and thankfully no longer has to worry about money. I just wish she didn't have to worry about me,' she said, touching a bottle. 'Which is why I'm so determined to turn things around. I need her to stop fretting about my dire financial situation.'

'I'm sorry things are so grim for you.' His hand rested over hers, and the sensation gave her quite a jolt. 'You don't deserve it. I hope this job makes things better for you.'

'Me too.' Her brain told her to move her hand, but for some reason her body wasn't cooperating. 'I can't fully move on until that wretched tax debt is cleared, but once that's sorted, I'm hoping I can make a fresh start and turn things around.'

She slid her hand out from underneath his. Touching him in such a confined space felt too intimate, even though she knew there was no ulterior motive. He wasn't that kind of man. And even if he was, he wouldn't be interested in her. He was a Ferrari; she was a 2CV.

'Talking of money,' she said, moving away in the guise of admiring the wine. 'I've listed the garage blocks for auction. That should free up some cash.'

He followed her around the confined space, flinching when he nearly collided with a cobweb. 'I thought we couldn't sell anything until probate had been granted?'

'Normally, we can't. But as the value of the estate is so large, we don't have the funds to pay Inheritance Tax, which has to be settled before the grant of probate can be issued.' She blew dust away from one of the labels. 'This wine is over eighty years old.'

'Some of them are even older.' He lifted a bottle from the rack. 'This one was bottled in 1901. So what do we do about the tax bill?'

'That's where Alex comes in. We can apply for an instalment option and delay paying Inheritance Tax, as long as we provide robust accounts. It'll buy you more time if you decide you want to continue running the place.'

'Which I don't.'

'No, but at least this way we can get probate granted and start selling off assets. Alex is meeting with the tax people tomorrow to formalise the application. I probably should've run it past you, but I knew you didn't have the funds to pay the Inheritance Tax upfront.'

'I don't, not unless I sell my house in Leeds.'

'You don't want to do that... do you?'

'Not really.' He replaced the wine bottle. 'Or at least, I didn't think I did. Truth is, I'm not sure I want to live there anymore.'

She glanced at him. 'Why's that?'

He shrugged. 'Bad memories. Maybe I'd be better of selling up and starting afresh somewhere else, like you're doing.' He shook his head. 'Anyway, I'm fine with your plan to arrange an instalment agreement. Thanks for doing that. I appreciate it.'

'No problem. Happy to help.'

His eyes met hers and when he spoke, his voice was barely a whisper. 'I don't know what I'd do without you.'

The small space seemed to close in on her. 'Not something you have to worry about. I'm not going anywhere,' she said, trying to keep her tone light, but it didn't stop the long pause that followed.

A pause in which they both looked at each other, unsure of what was happening... until a spider landed on Calvin's forehead and he nearly upended one of the wine racks in his attempt to escape it.

'Christ, get it off me!' he yelled, his usual calm demeanour suddenly gone.

'Stand still,' she said, trying to remove the spider, which was tricky since his arms were flailing about. 'I can't catch it unless you stay still.'

He calmed down to a degree, but he was still twitching. 'Has it gone?'

'It's gone,' she said, depositing the spider on the floor. 'Panic over.'

He swiped at his face. 'I can't stand creepy-crawlies.'

'You don't say?'

'Have you seen enough? Shall we head upstairs?' He was already backing towards the stairwell.

'Of course.' She followed him over to the steps. 'Now I know where the cellar is, I can arrange a proper valuation. Thanks for showing me around.'

'No problem.' He flinched when something touched his hair. 'After you.'

Kate headed up the steps, relieved that whatever had been crackling away between them had disappeared... courtesy of an interloping spider.

Chapter Ten

Wednesday, 8th December

As a footballer, Calvin was used to being at the receiving end of a team talk. Whether it was an analysis of a training session, or a half-time bollocking from the manager when the team were 3-0 down, he'd accept what was thrown at him – including a football boot once. It didn't matter whether you agreed with what was being said, or not. You learnt to keep your mouth shut, accept criticism and, crucially, never answer back.

But he wasn't used to leading the team. Or, in this case, the staff and residents of a care home. He'd never made captain at Leeds Park United, and although he'd tried to set a good example on the pitch, he'd never been the one formally at the helm. Until now.

He'd arranged this morning's meeting because decisions needed to be made about the care home's finances. And unlike football management, this required a collaborative approach. He wasn't equipped to make these decisions by himself.

All eyes were fixed on him as he stood by the dining-room doorway, his eager audience awaiting news of the future of the care home. He was feeling the pressure.

He'd scheduled the meeting first thing after breakfast, so Natalie could be included before she clocked off from her night shift. Her eyes were already drifting shut, not helped by Jacob asleep in her arms, willing his mum to join him in a nap.

The rest of the group were seated at small tables around the dining room, including Kate and Alex, who'd been persuaded to attend in case there were any questions that Calvin couldn't answer. They looked as apprehensive as he did.

He took a mouthful of water and cleared his throat. 'Thanks for coming, everyone. I wanted to give you an update on the care home's financial situation and allow you the opportunity to contribute to any discussions about what happens next. We currently have just over forty grand available to spend, which I'm proposing—'

'Where money come from?' Hanna's loud voice overrode his.

He looked over to see her scowling, her arms folded across her chest, her black eyeliner emphasising her steely glare.

Thankfully, he'd anticipated this question. 'I've been able to free up some funds ahead of probate being granted,' he said, unwilling to admit he'd resorted to cashing in his own personal shares in a Leeds–based clothing company, much against the advice of his accountant.

He tried not to catch Kate's eye, since he knew she would also be puzzled as to where the money had come from. But this was his decision, and he hadn't felt comfortable letting things carry on as they were.

'If money available, why not do it before?' Hanna looked daggers at him. 'Why wait until desperate times? You see how we suffer.' She gestured to the group, emphasising her point.

'The money has only just become available, Hanna. I assure you, if I'd had it any sooner, I would've told you. The question is, what do we do now we have it?'

'Pay staff,' Hanna said, as if it was obvious.

'I agree. But there's not enough to pay ongoing salaries, only the backdated pay owed for the last six months.'

'But not next month? Or month after?' Hanna's voice went up a notch. 'How we supposed to live?' She switched her glare in Alex's direction. 'Don't tell me rubbish about getting good deal staying here. Not good deal. Very *bad* deal.'

Alex cowered in his chair and tried to hide behind Kate, who didn't look any more comfortable than he did.

'It's better than nothing,' Natalie chipped in, rocking Jacob. 'I'd be very grateful to receive the money. Thank you, Calvin.'

Hanna raised her shoulders at Natalie, as if to say, *whatever*.

Calvin took a sip of water. 'That leaves us with approximately fifteen grand. I'd suggest we use twelve grand to clear the care home debts, pay this year's business rates and settle outstanding bills with our local suppliers in the village. I don't want to stretch their goodwill any further and risk them stopping supplying us.'

'But you happy to stretch *our* goodwill,' Hanna said, shaking her head.

'I think it's a great suggestion, Calvin.' Geraldine stroked a sleeping Suki, who was curled up by her feet. 'We can't afford to keep them waiting any longer. You have my vote.'

'Mine, too.' Natalie's agreement was followed by more murmuring and the raising of hands.

Hanna continued to scowl.

Calvin glanced over at Kate and she gave him a discreet thumbs up. It was a small gesture, but he was grateful nonetheless.

'That's settled then,' he said, forcing a smile, and praying for the day when this would be someone else's responsibility. 'That leaves us with about three grand, which is where you come in. The options, as I see it, are as follows. We could use the money to buy in external services, such as a locum nurse to cover a few shifts each week until the new year, when hopefully more funds will become available. Or we use the money to carry out maintenance repairs on the windows in the bedrooms, which keep banging open when it's windy.'

'Oh, that's not the wind,' Rowan said, adjusting his burgundy cravat. 'That's Ursula getting restless.' He looked up at the ceiling and wagged his finger. 'Naughty, Ursula.'

Kate's eyes drifted upwards, clearly perplexed as to why Rowan was talking to the ceiling. 'Er… who's Ursula?' she said, looking around the room.

'Ursula is the resident ghost,' Rowan said, turning to Kate. 'She's rather a minx. I've told her to pack it in on numerous occasions, but she does like to cause a stir. Only the other day she emptied the contents of my wardrobe and left all my waistcoats scattered across the floor, the brazen hussy.'

Esme reached across and patted his hand. 'That wasn't Ursula. That was your dementia.'

'I do not have dementia,' he said, haughtily. 'How very dare you.'

'Well, it's more plausible than a ghost emptying your wardrobe,' Esme said, looking both regal and festive in her emerald green dress and matching gold scarf.

'It's not just me she interacts with,' he said, pointing at Kate. 'Poor Kate was nearly tipped off the stepladders the other day when Ursula took umbrage at having a younger attractive female in the house. You can't tell me Kate is suffering from dementia.'

Kate flushed bright pink when everyone turned to look at her.

Calvin offered her a feeble smile, his attempt at an apology.

Esme placed her cup in its saucer. 'No, but Kate is suffering from extreme exhaustion, and regularly skips meals. So nearly falling off a ladder is hardly a shocking occurrence.'

'Excuse me, but I am sitting here,' an embarrassed-looking Kate said, clearly uncomfortable at having her mental wellbeing openly discussed.

Calvin could empathise; he wouldn't like that either.

He tried to bring things back on track. 'Regardless of whether the place is haunted,' he said, trying not to publicly accuse Rowan of being a fantasist, 'a number of windows are broken and need fixing.'

Lucky Larry raised his hand. 'If it was up to me, I'd be in favour of getting in help for Natalie and Hanna. The poor gals never get a break, and we'd be lost without them.'

Natalie mouthed, 'Thank you,' at Larry.

Hanna blew him a kiss. 'You family,' she said, fiercely. 'We not abandon you.'

Calvin might have been touched at seeing a softer side to the formidable nurse, if she hadn't then turned and glowered at him. He was just grateful she wasn't grumpy with the residents. She saved that side of her for him. And Alex, who'd also unwittingly been cast as a villain. Poor bloke.

'Is everyone in favour of hiring a locum nurse?' Calvin counted the hands that shot in the air. It was unanimous, supported by Deshad, who was watching the meeting via video link from upstairs. 'Great. I'll get on to that today.'

'Is there any news about what's happening with the care home, long term?' Geraldine asked, looking at the others. 'I think we're all keen to know what the future holds.'

Calvin took another sip of water, delaying answering so he could formulate a careful response. He needed to tread carefully, as he didn't want to upset anyone any sooner than he had to. 'Kate is making good progress with valuing the assets, and she's hoping to make the probate application before the end of the year. That's right, isn't it, Kate?'

He hoped she wouldn't object to being drawn into the conversation, but he needed an ally, and he knew she wouldn't throw him under the bus. How he knew this, he wasn't sure. It wasn't like he really knew her, but for some reason he trusted that she wouldn't shaft him by revealing the truth... namely, that he had every intention of selling up.

She stood up so everyone could see her. Her hair was fixed in a ponytail and her long hooded cardigan made her look like Little Red Riding Hood. Her attempts to remain invisible by tucking herself into the corner of the room had failed. Mostly because of him. He hoped she wouldn't hold that against him.

'I'm halfway through dealing with the ledgers,' she said, addressing the group nervously. 'So the list of assets is coming along nicely. We have a valuer from a local auction house visiting this afternoon, and he's going to catalogue the artwork and period furniture.'

'You're not planning on selling everything, are you?' An outraged Rowan turned to Calvin. 'Darling boy, you simply can't. Those pieces are part of the character of the house, they've been in the family for several centuries. Ursula would go berserk. She's one step away from turning into a poltergeist as it is, this could tip her over the edge.'

Calvin wasn't quite sure how to respond to that.

Thankfully, Kate came to his rescue. 'There are no immediate plans to sell anything, Rowan. This is purely an exercise in valuing the estate so that Inheritance Tax can be calculated. Something we're legally required to do before probate can be granted. The quicker we get this done, the sooner the care home can return to being a viable business. There's really no reason to worry,' she said, sharing a glance with Calvin. 'And I'm sure Calvin will give you plenty of notice before any firm decisions are made about the future of the care home.' She met his gaze. 'That's right, isn't it?'

He manged a feeble nod. 'Of course.' Swallowing awkwardly, he took another sip of water. 'Kate has listed my late uncle's garage blocks for auction this month, so that'll generate more income, which we can use to extend nursing cover. And Alex has done a great job getting to grips with the accounts and negotiating with our creditors. We're in a much better financial position than we were before they arrived. I'm grateful to them both.'

'Here, here,' Rowan said, starting off a round of applause, much to Kate's horror. She blushed and rapidly sat down, and Alex slid further down in his chair, both of them mortified at being the centre of attention.

Calvin glanced around the room and realised his granny was looking directly at him. She had a knowing smile that indicated trouble was looming. Her eyes drifted over to Kate, before coming back to land on him. What was she up to?

He cleared his throat and reached for his water; his mouth was bone dry again. 'That just leaves us with plans for

Christmas. There're a number of activities taking place in the village, so I'll put up a list in the foyer. If you could add your names to any events you're interested in attending, I'll book a minibus to take everyone.'

There was a general murmur of excitement.

'I do love Christmas,' Rowan said, clapping his hands. 'Such a fun time.'

'Me too.' Natalie looked lovingly down at her son. 'It'll be Jacob's first Christmas. I want to make it special for him.'

This was met with a smattering of *ahhhs*.

'Are we doing anything here at the care home?' Esme asked, her smile laced with mischief. She was up to something, he just knew it. 'I'm happy to organise a Secret Santa.'

'What is that?' Hanna's arms were still folded, but she looked less venomous than before. He was grateful for small mercies.

Esme turned to her. 'We put everyone's names into a hat, and then randomly select one person to buy a gift for. That way everyone gets a present, but it keeps the cost down.'

Hanna nodded. 'Good system. I like. But we all buy for baby, yes?'

'Oh, yes.' Esme looked at the others for confirmation. 'Absolutely.'

'Oh, please, I can't ask you to do that.' Natalie looked stricken. 'It's too much.'

'Not too much.' Hanna shook her head vehemently. 'Baby have no family to buy him presents. We buy presents instead. We baby's family.'

Natalie wiped her eyes. 'Thank you. That's so lovely of you. I'm more than happy to put up decorations, if that helps.'

'I can help with that, too.' Kate raised her hand, as if she were in school. 'I like putting up decorations.' She blushed when Calvin looked at her.

He was touched by her willingness to join in with the festivities. It certainly wasn't part of her job remit.

'And I'm happy to arrange a film night,' Rowan said, waving theatrically. '*White Christmas* is an absolute must.'

Esme gave him a pointed look. 'As long as it's not *The Nightmare Before Christmas*. Or *Die Hard*.'

'*Die Hard* isn't a Christmas film,' Larry said, shaking his head. 'I'll defy anyone who tells me otherwise.'

Rowan let out a theatrical sigh. 'Credit me with some taste, darlings. If it doesn't contain music composed by Irving Berlin or Stephen Sondheim then it won't make the cut.'

'That's my Christmas ruined,' Geraldine said, drily.

'What's that, Ursula…?' Rowan stared up at the ceiling. 'Yes, of course we'll include *Miracle on 34th Street*… and, yes, the original, not the remake,' he said, rolling his eyes, as if the demands of the care home's resident ghost were draining his patience. 'Such a drama queen.'

Kate smothered a laugh. The irony wasn't lost on Calvin either.

'Put me down in charge of music,' Larry said, glancing at Geraldine. 'I'm happy to take requests.'

Geraldine beamed. 'Bless you. At least I can be assured of one tasteful evening… And where are you off to?' Suki had got up and walked over to Calvin, plonking herself down by his feet. Geraldine's hands went to her hips. 'Oh, like that, is it?'

Calvin shrugged an apology and slid his feet from underneath the dog.

'I can sort out a quiz… if you like,' a tentative voice called from the back.

All heads turned to see who had spoken.

Geraldine strained her head. 'Who said that?'

'Me.' Alex stood briefly, and then immediately sat back down again.

Calvin gave him a thumbs up. 'Thanks, Alex. Sounds like we have everything sorted.' He looked around the room. 'Is there anything else anyone wants to raise before we finish?'

'Yes, I do.' Geraldine struggled to her feet. 'I think I speak for everyone when I say how grateful we are to have you here, Calvin.'

His insides squirmed. 'There's no need, Geraldine—'

'Yes, there is.' She raised her hand to stop him. 'I know things aren't perfect, and we still have a heap of problems to overcome, but we'd be in a much worse state if you hadn't shown up. No one was forcing you to stay here and deal with us lot. You could've easily buggered off back to Leeds and left us to it, but you didn't. You've worked your socks off trying to make things better for us, and we're very grateful... even if we don't act like it sometimes.'

'Here, here!' Rowan started clapping, encouraging everyone else to join in.

Calvin's mortification hiked up another notch. He wanted the ground to open and swallow him up.

Geraldine bundled into him and clasped his face in her hands. He had a horrible feeling he knew what was coming next. 'Your uncle would be so proud of the way you've stepped up. You're a credit to him.' She kissed him. Of course she did, why was he even surprised.

Aside from the humiliation of being kissed in public by a woman old enough to be his grandmother, it was hearing everyone's cheering and thank yous that unsettled him most. Even the dog had joined in. Suki jumped up and licked his hand, her tail wagging furiously.

Guilt flooded through him. He felt like such a fraud.

They were thanking him for staying... when all he wanted to do was run away.

They thought he was a decent bloke... when he was anything but.

They were expecting miracles and the care home to be saved. When in reality he had no intention of saving anything.

Once probate was granted, he was off. Back to Leeds. His family, his friends. His old life. He wasn't some kind-hearted saviour. He was a failed footballer with nothing to offer these people except momentary respite from the inevitable. They deserved better.

He didn't think anything could make him feel worse, until he saw the look on Granny Esme's face. Pride, mixed in with hope, and a dash of misguided belief that he might be softening to the idea of staying.

Christ, he hated letting people down.

Chapter Eleven

Friday, 10th December

Kate couldn't remember the last time she'd travelled in a minibus. It was probably the school trip she'd gone on, to Wales, as a kid. A trip that her aunt and uncle had paid for, which had inadvertently upset her mum. Not that her mum had ever said anything, but Kate knew she'd wanted to pay for the excursion herself – she just couldn't afford it.

Today's outing reminded Kate of that noisy and boisterous road trip. Only, instead of a bunch of unruly teenagers causing mayhem, it was the care home residents and staff playing up... except for Hanna, who'd stayed behind to look after Priya.

Alex had also declined to attend Pluckley's Christmas lights switch-on event, preferring to stay in and watch TV. Although, how much peace and quiet he'd get, Kate wasn't sure. As they'd loaded everyone into the minibus, ready to depart, a moped had pulled up and handed Alex a takeaway pizza, much to the disgust of Hanna, who had accused him of being selfish, as he hadn't ordered her one. As the bus had pulled away, all Kate could see when she glanced back was the pair of them arguing on the care-home steps – with Alex trying to hand over his pizza to Hanna, and Hanna making a show of refusing.

Things weren't a lot calmer in the minibus. Natalie was trying to pacify a crying Jacob, Geraldine was giving Calvin instructions on how to drive the bus, and Rowan and Esme were knocking back the contents of a hip flask. Judging by their rosy cheeks and raucous laughter, Kate suspected their claim of it containing 'hot chocolate' was stretching the truth somewhat. If it *was* hot chocolate, then it was laced with something a lot stronger.

Any hope Kate had of remaining inconspicuous, tucked away at the back of the bus, vanished when Rowan turned to her. 'I hear Ursula's been up to her old tricks. Rumour has it she hid your drinking glass and stole your pen.'

Nothing remained private at the care home, Kate had discovered. 'Correction: I *lost* my pen, and someone probably moved my drinking glass when they were tidying up. No doubt I left it somewhere when I was showing the auctioneer around,' she said, trying not to encourage Rowan in his fantasies.

She'd had a manic few days, dealing with the representative from the auction house and trying to agree lease values for the properties in London. Getting flustered and mislaying things had been inevitable, as her focus was all over the place. She wasn't about to let Rowan attribute it to the actions of a random ghost. She was struggling to hold on to her sanity as it was.

Rowan tapped his lip in contemplation. 'I still believe it was Ursula, up to her tricks. Was the pen of sentimental value?'

Kate shrugged. 'Kind of.' It had been a graduation present from her mum, but she didn't want to give Rowan any further ammunition.

'That's her modus operandi, discovering what a person cares about and torturing them by stealing it. She's quite the minx.' Rowan reached over and patted her hand. 'Talking of spirit connections, you might want to avoid the churchyard tonight. If you think Ursula is a tricky customer, heaven only knows how you'll react if you encounter the Red Lady.'

'Rowan, can you stop scaring Kate, please?' Calvin shouted from the front of the minibus. 'This is supposed to be a fun night out.'

Kate caught Calvin's expression in the rear-view mirror and saw his exaggerated eye-roll. She couldn't help smiling.

Unfortunately, Rowan wasn't to be deterred and leant closer, lowering his voice. 'The Red Lady is a sorrowing ghost who wanders mournfully through the graveyard, searching for the body of her baby, who lies somewhere in an unmarked grave.'

Esme made a spooky ghost noise, which made Kate laugh.

Rowan tutted disapprovingly and turned to glare at her. 'Do you mind?'

'I was just adding some atmosphere,' Esme said, her speech slightly slurred from the amount of 'hot chocolate' she'd drunk.

'I don't need any help, thank you, darling.' He turned back to Kate. 'The Red Lady was a member of the Dering family and thought to have died in childbirth. Why the offspring to such a notable family should lie away from the family vault in some unmarked spot is unknown. But it could be that the child died before there was a chance for it to be baptised, meaning a Christian burial could've been denied.'

The minibus jolted as they drove over a pothole, causing Geraldine to moan at Calvin for not avoiding it and Jacob to increase the intensity of his crying.

Annoyed at having his flow interrupted, Rowan refocused. 'The churchyard is hallowed ground and in some eyes the child's body would have had no right to be there, but his mother still searches for him, night after night, calling to her lost child.'

Kate supressed a sigh. 'Why is she called the Red Lady?'

'No one is entirely sure,' he said, excited by her question. 'It could be the colour of the gown she wears, or maybe her hair. But a ghostly red hue can be seen drifting through the gravestones, visible only to those with a spiritual connection… like you,' he said, patting her hand. 'And me, of course.' He wasn't about to be outdone.

'I'll be sure to let you know if I see her, Rowan.'

'Please do! It would make my night. My year, even.'

Thankfully, they arrived at the village square and Calvin parked up.

He helped everyone off the bus, appearing by Kate's side a moment later. 'What are the chances of those two remaining sober?' he said, as Esme and Rowan swayed towards The Black

Horse Inn and joined in with the carollers, who were belting out 'O, Holy Night' in front of the church entrance.

'Slim-to-none,' she said, smiling. 'We may need wheelchairs to get them home.'

'Already thought of that.' He pointed to the boot of the minibus. 'But I only have two!' he called out to the retreating group, which included Geraldine and Lucky Larry, as they also made a beeline for the pub. 'The rest of you need to retain the use of your legs!'

Laughing, Kate zipped up her coat. 'They're not interested in the lights switch-on at all, are they?'

'Nope. They just wanted an excuse for a booze-up.'

'And I thought he was going to cause the most trouble tonight,' Natalie said, placing Jacob in his pushchair. 'You've got competition, Jacob.' She tucked in his blanket. 'I'll take him for a stroll and see if he'll settle. Have a good night, both of you,' she said, heading towards the carol singers.

Calvin watched them for a moment, his expression concerned. 'She looks tired.'

Kate slipped on her gloves, as it was a chilly night. 'Any luck getting a locum nurse?'

'I've registered with a couple of agencies. Hopefully, we can get someone soon.'

'It's a shame she doesn't have anyone to help her.' Kate searched for her scarf, wondering if she'd left it on the minibus. 'I'm guessing her family don't live close by?'

'I've no idea,' he said, with a shrug. 'She doesn't talk about them. All I know is that she was made homeless when her husband filed for divorce and she was forced to vacate the military property she lived in.'

'Seems a bit harsh.'

'Especially as he's serving abroad at the moment. The property's sitting empty… What are you looking for?'

'My scarf.'

Calvin smiled. 'You mean, the scarf you're already wearing?'

Surely not? She touched her neck, only to feel soft wool. It was official: she was losing her mind. 'Don't say a word.'

'Wouldn't dream of it.' Suppressing his grin, he pointed to a row of stalls set up outside the village shops. 'Mulled wine? Mince pie?'

As she looked over, it occurred to her that it was just the two of them left – everyone else had disappeared. She wasn't sure how she felt about that. 'Yes, okay… but I could do with proper food first. I skipped dinner and I'm starving.'

'You also skipped lunch.'

She folded her arms. 'What are you, the food police? Anyway, I didn't skip lunch, I had crisps.'

'Crisps are not lunch. And they're not healthy.'

She shook her head. 'You sound like my mum.'

'Good. Then maybe you'll listen to me… Katiekins.' He steered her towards the food stalls.

She laughed, even though she wasn't sure about being called 'Katiekins' by anyone other than her mum. Nonetheless, she allowed him to lead her over to a stall selling hot food – she was too hungry to argue. 'What's your nickname?' she asked, needing to redress the balance.

'Don't have one.' He pointed to the menu board. 'What do you fancy?'

'All footballers have nicknames.' She read the list of options. They had everything from hot dogs to melted-brie-and-cranberry toasties. Her stomach growled appreciatively.

He was standing next to her, looking fashionably warm in his layered outfit of brown jacket over a green hoodie. 'Know a lot about being a footballer, do you?'

'I know enough.' She glanced up, noticing the way his hair was tucked through the gap of his baseball cap. 'What was it? Johno? Jonnyboy? Boris?'

He laughed. 'None of the above. I told you, I don't have a nickname.'

'I don't believe you.' She returned to studying the menu. 'I'll find out, you know.'

'No, you won't. Now concentrate.' He pointed to the menu board. 'What do you want?'

'Chilli, please.'

He dug out his wallet. 'I'm paying for this, so don't even bother arguing.'

'Fine.' She rolled her eyes. 'Thank you. You can deduct it from my bill.' She ignored the look he shot her. Behind them a group of people had congregated on a makeshift stage. 'What does your mum call you?'

For a moment she didn't think he was going to answer, but then he said, 'My family call me Cal.' He turned away to order the food.

Kate watched the activity taking place on the stage. A man was tapping a microphone, and a plump Father Christmas was entertaining the kids congregated below. The village square was packed with people milling about, enjoying the festive atmosphere. It was a heart-warming sight.

'Here you go.' Calvin handed her a carton, complete with plastic fork and festive napkins.

The chilli smelt fantastic. She took a mouthful, sucking in cool air when she realised it was hot. 'Aren't you having anything?'

'Maybe later. I've already eaten.' He watched her eat. 'Good?'

'Really good.'

'Is your appetite improving?'

'Yes, thanks.' She ate some more. 'This is delicious.'

He seemed to study her. 'Then how come you still skip meals?'

She lifted her shoulders. 'Too busy, I guess. Before I didn't eat because I didn't want to. Now it's because I get engrossed in what I'm doing and forget. Usually, Geraldine or Esme bring me something if they know I haven't eaten, so I'm never going to starve.'

He rubbed his forehead. 'You need to take regular breaks, Kate. I don't want you working yourself into the ground. Or, you know… having a panic attack.' He'd lowered his voice, as if fearful of being overheard.

'Well, neither do I, but I'm hoping they've stopped,' she replied, embarrassed at the mention of her fragile state of mind – not that she could blame him. After all, she was the woman who hadn't realised she was already wearing her scarf. 'Or at least, they've reduced. They don't happen every day now.' She moved away from the food stalls. 'Let's head over, ready for the lights switch-on.'

He followed her towards the main square. 'Have you spoken to anyone about it?'

She shook her head. 'It's not like I don't know the cause.'

'Still, you should seek professional help.'

She stopped to face him. 'Oh, you mean like you have for dealing with your HMC?'

'HCM.'

'Whatever. I don't see you seeking professional help.' She resumed eating, hoping he'd take the hint and quit talking about it.

'I don't have panic attacks,' he said, barely audible above the noise of the carol singers, who were now belting out 'Joy to the World'.

She was about to argue, when she saw the pained expression on his face and her annoyance melted away. 'Doesn't mean you're okay,' she said, softly.

His gaze dropped to his feet. 'Why do you think I'm not okay? I'm fine.'

'Are you? Because most people wouldn't be.'

Her dad certainly hadn't been. He'd struggled with his demons, and look how that had ended. She'd hate for Calvin to head down the same slippery path.

The man on stage approached the microphone and announced that the countdown had started for the lights switch-on. 'TEN!' He gestured for everyone to join in. 'NINE!'

'The way I see it, I've just got to get on with it.' Calvin turned to the stage. 'Talking about it won't help.'

'EIGHT… SEVEN!'

Kate glanced up at him, hating to see such sadness etched on his face. 'In which case, you need to find another way of dealing with your loss, so you can move on.' She turned away and joined in with the countdown. 'FOUR… THREE!'

A few seconds later, everyone cheered and the village square burst into a sparkle of flashing lights. The giant Christmas tree glowed with silver stars, illuminating the reindeer positioned around its base. The carollers began to sing 'We Wish You a Merry Christmas' and everyone joined in. Children danced around, couples held hands, and a group of young lads held their beers aloft and toasted the festivities.

They'd certainly never had anything like this in Clapham. It was nice being part of a community event. She glanced across at Calvin, realising this was probably what he missed about playing football, that sense of being part of a team.

She closed the lid on her empty chilli carton and nudged him. 'What about hobbies? What interests do you have? You know, aside from football.'

He looked surprised by her question. 'I don't have anything in my life aside from football.' He gave a half-hearted shrug. 'Other than my family.'

'Then no wonder you're so depressed,' she said, heading for a bin at the side of the square.

He caught up with her. 'I'm not depressed.'

She binned the carton. 'Grief-stricken, then. Whatever you want to call it.'

'Taking up a hobby isn't going to change that.'

'How do you know if you've never tried?' She walked off, glancing back. 'Time for mulled wine. You coming?'

He jogged to catch her up. 'Have you always had hobbies?'

She wrapped her scarf tighter. 'Music, mainly. I wouldn't have got through the last few years without it. It was the only thing keeping me sane.'

He sidestepped a group of kids playing with sparklers. 'How come?'

She thought about it. 'It relaxes me, I guess. Stops me overthinking and erases any negative thoughts I might be having. Music is known to release mood-enhancing endorphins, you know... like eating, exercising and having...' She trailed off, suddenly feeling like an awkward teenager discussing sex with a parent. 'Er... well, you know... falling in love.' Flustered, she avoided looking at him until they arrived at the food stalls, where she hastily ordered two mulled wines. 'My turn to get these.'

He resisted saying anything and allowed her to pay. 'How did you get into music? Did you learn to play as a kid?'

She handed him his warm drink. 'I started with the guitar. My dad used to play, so I guess it's in the genes. I went through a stage of wanting to feel closer to him, so Mum gave me his old acoustic guitar. We had a neighbour who played, so he taught me a few chords in exchange for me mowing his lawn.' She sipped her mulled wine; it was warm and spicy, and made her tongue tingle. 'Then one Christmas my aunt and uncle bought my cousins a piano. They showed absolutely no interest in playing it and moaned about having lessons, so in the end I was given the lessons instead.'

He sipped his wine. 'How did your mum feel about that? I remember you saying she was sensitive about money.'

'Well remembered.' She almost laughed at his expression, as he swallowed his wine. 'How's your mulled wine?'

'Sweet,' he said, pulling a face.

She cupped her hands around the warm cup. 'You're right, it did cause a problem. For a long while I kept quiet and didn't tell her. I really wanted the lessons, but I knew if she found out, she'd insist on paying and she couldn't afford it.'

He took another sip of wine and grimaced. 'I'm guessing she found out eventually?'

'She wasn't happy, but in the end we came to an agreement. I'd keep having the lessons, but they'd be instead of birthday and Christmas presents... You're really not enjoying that, are you?' She turned to the stallholder and ordered him a beer.

'You don't have to do that,' he said, trying to stop her. 'It's fine.'

'It's not fine. Admit it, you hate it?'

He attempted to argue, but then shrugged. 'Okay, you win. It's disgusting. But make it a light beer – I'm driving, remember? Geraldine is critical enough as it is.'

Kate paid the stallholder. 'Geraldine will be too pissed to notice.'

He laughed and she felt a rush of pure relief at seeing his face brighten. Sadness really didn't suit him.

He binned his wine and accepted the beer. 'So you never had presents?'

'Not from the age of twelve onwards, no. Mum would get me a little gift to open, so I always had something. I didn't mind, I loved music that much.'

He took a swig of beer. 'Do you still play?'

'Not as much as I'd like. I don't have my instruments anymore.' Her chest twinged as the loss hit her once again. She missed playing so much. Maybe that's why her anxiety levels had increased? She had nothing to diffuse it and balance out the negativity filling her head.

He was frowning. 'What about the piano I saw at your flat?'

'I had nowhere to store it,' she said, swallowing past the tightness in her throat. 'And I couldn't afford the fees for professional storage, so I gave it away to a kid who wanted to play but couldn't afford an instrument of his own. It's gone to a good home.' She distracted herself by drinking more wine, hoping for an anaesthetic to quell the pain. It hadn't been an expensive piano, but it had been hers, and it had given her hours of pleasure. Parting with it had been a wrench. 'How's your beer?'

'Good, thanks.'

'Shall we walk up to the main square?'

'Sure.' He waited until they had escaped the crowds, before asking, 'What about your dad's guitar? What happened to that?'

Kate stared straight ahead. 'My ex-husband sold it,' she said, unsurprised by the wobble in her voice. It never got any easier to say.

Calvin abruptly stopped and caught her arm. 'He did what?'

Reluctantly, she turned to face him. 'You don't need to say it, okay? Believe me, I'm painfully aware of how awful it is. It was a special anniversary edition, so it was worth quite a bit of money, and Tristan was… well, he was desperate and in a bad way, and I don't know… Desperate people do desperate things. He needed the money.'

'That's no excuse.' The warmth of Calvin's hand squeezing her arm threatened to undo her.

She forced away the sadness, in case she had another melt-down. 'You're right, I know.' She knocked back the rest of her mulled wine and binned the cup, needing a moment to compose herself. 'Can we explore the church while we're here?'

He must have sensed she needed to switch topic. 'Are you sure? You're not put off by Rowan's scary stories?'

She gave him what she hoped was an admonishing look. 'Rowan's stories are not scary, they're delusional. And besides, you said you didn't believe in ghosts.'

'I don't. Doesn't mean I don't jump when I watch a horror movie.'

'Then why watch them?' She'd never understood how people could enjoy being scared witless.

'The rush, I suppose.' He nodded towards the church. 'Are we doing this?'

She nodded assertively. 'We are.'

They left the main square and walked past the flashing Christmas tree, looking resplendent as it twinkled away. Nestled between the garden of The Black Horse Inn and a row of olde-worlde cottages was a wide footpath leading up to St Nicholas's church. The intense darkness that shrouded them as they headed towards the graveyard was interspersed by the festive lights decorating the quaint country cottages.

Directly ahead, the church's grounds stretched into the distance, the sombre space awash with shadows and tombstones, lit by the occasional solar light buried into the ground.

Kate studied the landscape, aware that the noise from tonight's event had been replaced by an eerie silence. 'These headstones are so old, the inscriptions have faded,' she said, using the torch on her phone to illuminate the writing. 'No sign of the Red Lady, though.' Her smile faded when she turned and was greeted by an empty pathway. 'Calvin?'

He stepped out from behind a tombstone. 'Yes?'

Relief flooded her. 'I couldn't see where you were.'

He walked towards her, grinning. 'Not scared, were you?'

'Of course not,' she scoffed, attempting to hide her jumpiness.

He pointed to the church. 'Shall we go inside?'

'Will it be open at this time of night?'

'Only one way to find out.'

They continued down the pathway, which circled the church, bringing them round to the main entrance. A stone archway led up to a large wooden door.

Calvin opened the door and disappeared inside. 'We're in luck.'

Kate followed, stunned by what she saw.

The entire space was lit by huge candles sitting on top of ornate brass holders. The stone walls were painted white, and stained-glass windows led the eye up to a wooden domed ceiling. The cobbled flooring was uneven to walk on, and wooden carvings gave the pews a grandness that matched the plaques hanging from the walls, detailing historic events dating back to the sixteenth century.

'It's quite something, isn't it?' Kate made her way down the central aisle, heading towards an enclosed chapel at the end. As she ducked under the gold velvet curtain draped across the entrance, a flash of red skimmed past her eyeline, glittering as it passed through the light shining in from the small window above.

Calvin's sudden appearance through the doorway startled her. 'Everything okay?'

'All good,' she said, feigning a smile. But when she glanced down, she saw a scatter of red rose petals lying on the floor. She looked around, but there were no flowers on display. How odd.

'The church was built in the thirteenth century,' he said, picking up a pamphlet. 'By the monks of Canterbury on the site of a tenth-century Saxon church. It says there are two resident ghosts, the Red Lady, who you know about, and the White Lady.'

'Not very original with their names, are they?' She moved away from the chapel, deciding it would be sensible to stay closer to Calvin. Maybe her mind wouldn't play tricks on her and imagine things, if she wasn't alone.

'The White Lady was said to be the wife of a local lord,' he continued, holding the pamphlet under the candlelight to read. 'She was a lady of exquisite beauty and when she died tragically at an early age, her husband was so grief-stricken he sought a way to preserve her beauty forever.'

As she glanced at the text, her body brushed against his, absorbing a waft of his aftershave. She moved away. There was staying close, and then there was being *too* close. 'Sounds creepy.'

'Her body was sealed in a series of airtight glass coffins and placed in an open casket. She was laid to rest in the family crypt, where her beloved husband could continue to admire her beauty throughout his life.'

'A bit Norman Bates.'

Calvin smiled. 'Maybe he was trying to be romantic.'

'Well, he failed. Admiring your dead wife's body as she rots in a coffin is not romantic.'

'When you put it like that, I guess not.' Calvin returned to reading. 'Secure against the ravages of time the elaborate coffin may be, but it has not proved capable of restraining her restless spirit. In the still of night, she breaks free from the confines of the casket and wanders through the chapel, scattering rose petals – a single red rose clutched to her chest – as beautiful in death as she was in life.' When he looked up, his smile faded. 'What?'

Kate tried to exhale, but the air had got stuck in her lungs. *A red rose?*

When she started feeling dizzy, she knew she needed to sit down, before she embarrassed herself by fainting.

As gracefully as she could, she slid onto one of the wooden pews and rested her forehead on her hands. There was no such thing as ghosts. Seeing random red lights and stepping on rose petals was in no way evidence of ethereal beings. The light was probably a reflection of the festive lights outside. And the rose petals…?

'Are you okay?' He slid in next to her and placed his arm around her. She wasn't entirely sure whether this was a comfort, or a hindrance. 'Are you having a panic attack?'

She shook her head. She wasn't having a meltdown; she was simply hallucinating. *Was that better, or worse?* she wondered.

'Talk to me,' he said, rubbing her back, which had a strange effect on her breathing. 'I'm worried about you.'

She sat up and opened her eyes, intending to dismiss her crazy thoughts and not admit to having a wobble, when she spotted something in his hand. 'What's that?'

He lifted the silk scarf for her to see – a silk scarf that was decorated with red rose petals. 'I found it on the floor. Someone obviously dropped it, so I was going to leave it by the door in case they came back for it.'

Kate started laughing. She wasn't going mad. She hadn't imagined seeing the petals of the White Lady's red rose scattered across the floor; she'd simply seen a discarded scarf lying there and her idiotic brain had jumped to a whole host of implausible conclusions. She was officially a basket case.

'What's so funny?' Calvin's expression indicated that her slightly hysterical laughter was as alarming as her erratic breathing.

'Nothing, I'm fine. Really. A momentary blip.' As her lungs expelled the air and her body relaxed, the tension left her, and once again she felt herself slumping. Only this time, she ended up leaning against Calvin, her head nestled in the crook of his neck, her arm lying across his lap, her fingers entwined with his.

For a second, it didn't seem real. Like it was another hallucination, and she allowed herself a moment to enjoy the way he felt against her, warm and solid. His skin was soft, a contrast to the firm muscle beneath. And boy, did he smell good – of candles, mulled wine and a hint of beer.

And then reality came screeching into focus. This was not some imaginary dream, or a moment of secret fantasy, fuelled by wishful thinking. She really was slumped across Calvin Johnson, her nose pressed against his smooth skin, breathing him in as she softly moaned. *Oh, good lord!*

She wasn't sure who froze first – her or him.

There was a moment of absolute stillness, followed by a stiffening of bodies, and then an awkward uncoupling, with both of them flustered and scrabbling to their feet.

'I'm so sorry,' she said, tripping over the kneeling cushion in her haste to escape. 'I don't know what came over me.'

'Not a problem,' he said, exiting the opposite end of the pew at such speed, it was obvious he couldn't get away fast enough.

'Time to get back to the minibus, I think.' She ran for the door.

'Absolutely,' he said, following her.

Just when she thought she couldn't possibly humiliate herself any more…

Chapter Twelve

Monday, 13th December

It was still dark when Calvin came downstairs, ready for his early-morning run. The thick fog that had descended yesterday had yet to clear and the low cloud shrouded the care home in a spooky mist. It looked like the setting for a supernatural horror film. Rowan would love it.

As he walked across the lobby, he was surprised to find Alex standing in front of the events noticeboard. 'You're up early, Alex. Everything okay?'

Alex gave a half-hearted shrug, his focus fixated on the noticeboard. 'Hanna wants help changing the slide-sheets this morning. It's a two-person job, apparently.'

Calvin frowned. 'It's not your responsibility to carry out care-home chores, Alex. Why didn't she ask Natalie to help? Or me, for that matter?'

'Natalie needs to look after Priya and everyone else is busy doing other stuff. Besides, saying no to Hanna comes with consequences.' He shot Calvin a look. 'Know what I mean?'

'Only too well. But I don't appreciate her bullying you into helping.'

'If I help her, she might stop yelling at me.'

Calvin rested his hand on Alex's shoulder. 'We've all been in Hanna's bad books at some point.'

Alex pointed to the noticeboard. 'And now I've got to buy her a Christmas present. What the hell am I going to get her?'

Calvin looked at the list of names pinned to the board. They'd been put into pairs, buying a present for one another.

So much for it being a secret draw. He searched for his name, unsurprised to see he'd been paired with Kate. Esme was scheming. He'd be having words with his granny.

'I'd better go and find Hanna,' Alex said, with a sigh, heading upstairs. 'She'll only come looking for me otherwise. See you later.'

'Good luck.' He wasn't comfortable with Hanna using Alex, but she didn't have many other people to ask and the locum wasn't in place yet. As talking to her was likely to make things worse, he'd be better off keeping quiet. Still, if she continued to abuse Alex's good nature, he might have to step in.

He made his way into the dining room and headed for the kitchen. Suki greeted him before he'd even reached the door. She came bounding over, her floppy blonde hair flying about as she jumped up and tried to lick him. He ruffled her ears, stupidly buoyed at being shown such affection – even if it was from a daft dog. 'Hey, there, girl. You ready for our run?'

'Not with this hip,' Granny Esme said, startling him.

He turned to see her sitting at the breakfast table, sipping a cup of coffee. 'You made me jump. How come you're up so early?'

'The curse of old age, an inability to sleep.' She was fully dressed, her navy jumpsuit teamed with a tartan shawl.

He frowned. 'Do you need to see a doctor?'

'It's nothing painkillers and a shot of brandy won't cure.' She gave him a sly grin. 'Where did you head off to yesterday? You were gone most of the day.'

Calvin checked the coast was clear before answering. He didn't want Geraldine overhearing. 'I went to meet with a representative from a national care-home company. They're interested in taking over the place.'

Esme lowered her coffee. 'You've made up your mind then? You're selling?'

'Nothing's decided,' he said, weighed down by the stress of it all. 'But I need to consider my options. How can I make an informed decision if I don't have all the facts? I needed to know more about how they operate.'

'And what did you discover?'

He considered her question. 'They're very professional, structured, and they have a solid business model. The literature is impressive, and I have no doubt they'd manage the place with integrity and make a decent profit.'

'So why the long face?'

'I'm not sure. It sounded perfect.' He stroked Suki's head, smiling into her huge brown eyes. It'd been a while since anyone had looked at him with such affection. Sad that it was a dog that was making eyes at him and not a human being. 'A bit too perfect.'

'Meaning?'

'I can't imagine they'd allow Deshad to stay, or Natalie to continue looking after Jacob, along with working full-time. Their approach seemed very formal and rigid, which is probably a good thing and what this place needs, but...' He sighed. 'I don't know... it felt a bit clinical and impersonal.'

His grandmother drank another mouthful of coffee. 'Then you have some more thinking to do.'

'Except I need to make a decision soon. I can't keep stringing everyone along, especially as Kate is close to finalising the probate application.'

'Quite the conundrum.' Esme studied him. 'Talking of Kate, the pair of you looked a little flustered over the weekend. Is everything okay?'

Trust Esme to notice.

'It's fine,' he lied, making a fuss of Suki, hoping to cover his embarrassment.

Friday night's lights switch-on event had been an evening of contrasting emotions. Part fun, part revelation – and ending in total confusion when she'd... well, he wasn't sure what had happened. One moment they were sitting on a pew, chatting, after she'd come over faint, and the next she was pressed against him, her face buried into his neck and softly moaning.

The most alarming aspect was his reaction. Instead of recoiling, he'd had an overwhelming urge to wrap his arms around her and... well, again, he wasn't sure what. All he knew was that he hadn't wanted it to end, which only made his mortification worse when she'd come to her senses, sprung away from him and run from the church, mumbling and apologising. He never got the chance to tell her that he hadn't minded, that he'd quite liked it and she had nothing to be sorry for.

But admitting that would only have complicated things further. So maybe it was better he hadn't said anything.

'Only, I saw her this morning,' Esme said, interrupting his thoughts. 'She looked rather upset.'

'Upset?'

'She came downstairs sniffing back tears and disappeared out the front door without a word. I wondered if something had happened between you two? An argument perhaps? Lovers' tiff?'

'Hardly. We work together, Granny... sorry, Esme.' He tried to cover his discomfort. 'When was this? Do you know where she went?'

'No idea.' Esme checked her watch. 'It was about twenty minutes ago.' Her gaze turned inquisitive. 'Only, it seemed like the pair of you were getting along rather well?' She tried and failed to make it sound like an innocent remark and not a probing question.

Thankfully, Geraldine appeared from the kitchen.

'Here's her lead,' she said, clipping it onto Suki's collar and handing him a bag of treats. 'Be a good girl for Calvin. Not that you take any notice of me anymore, do you?' Her eyes lifted to Calvin. 'You've stolen her heart, you bad man. Although I really can't blame her. She's not the only female falling for your charms.'

'Not just female,' Esme said, smiling. 'Rowan's a bit smitten, too.'

Both women laughed and Calvin decided it was time to escape. 'On that note, I'm off. See you later, ladies.'

'Bye!' they chorused, waving him off.

Securing his baseball hat in place, he headed outside to his car, Suki trotting obediently by his side. *What had happened to upset Kate?* he wondered. And so early in the day. He hoped it wasn't Rowan's scary ghost stories that had unsettled her.

Suki looked up with a puzzled expression when he opened the car door. 'In case we see Kate,' he said, as if the dumb dog would understand him. 'She might need a lift.'

With a resigned shake of the head, Suki jumped into the car, positioning herself on the front seat. He wasn't sure whether he was supposed to put a seatbelt on her, or not. She sat upright, head high, looking quite regal as she perused her surroundings.

'Don't get used to it,' he said, climbing in next to her. 'You'll be in the back later. I'm not having your muddy paws on my leather seats.'

She gave him a contemptuous glare and turned to look out the window – such was his relationship with females.

Heading away from the care home, he kept his eyes peeled for signs of Kate. Surely she wasn't still upset about Friday night? He hadn't seen much of her over the weekend but, other than being a bit embarrassed, he hadn't got the impression she was too traumatised. They'd had a couple of brief conversations, mainly about work stuff, but perhaps he should have reassured her it wasn't a big deal. Maybe she was worried he'd got the wrong idea, and was stressing over it?

He drove twice around the village, looking for her, struggling to see through the dense fog, but there were no signs of Kate.

Suki was getting fidgety, and he realised the poor animal probably needed a wee.

Turning into the lay-by next to Screaming Woods, he parked up and killed the engine.

'Keep an eye out for Kate,' he said, feeling a tad guilty for abandoning his search. He glanced at Suki, who tilted her head as if to say, 'I'm a dog, you stupid human.'

'Well, that's debatable,' he said, exiting the car and heading around to the passenger side.

Visibility was poor. The fog obscured the lane, making it precarious to cross the road. The other side wasn't much better. The trees had lost their foliage, making the dark trunks and branches merge into the mist.

'Don't run off,' he instructed Suki, unclipping her lead. 'Stay close.'

He was subjected to another look.

'I'm just saying.' He stretched out his hamstrings. 'I don't have time to go looking for you.' He broke into a jog. 'Come on, keep up.'

But Suki had disappeared into the bushes, no doubt keen to relieve herself.

Calvin set his watch and settled into a steady jog. The air was damp and the terrain underfoot uneven, covered with fallen branches and low-growing ferns. His mind kept drifting to thoughts of Kate and whether she was okay. She'd openly admitted she was still struggling. Should he call someone? Alex, maybe? Supposing something happened to her?

A few moments later, Suki caught up with him and they ran together through the wood, their breath visible against the cold December air.

He wasn't sure whether thoughts of Kate had conjured her up, or whether he'd started hallucinating, but a flash of red caught his eye and he ground to a halt. He turned sharply, recognising her long cardigan.

She looked to be embroiled in an argument with a tree. She was yelling at the large oak, hitting it with a thick branch, sending chunks of bark flying and knocking herself off balance in the process.

And then she disappeared from view.

He sprinted towards where she'd landed, fearful she'd injured herself. 'Kate! Are you okay? Where are you?'

He spotted her red cardigan and ran over, the dog not far behind.

She was lying face down, her hands bunched into fists, her feet kicking the ground like a toddler having a massive tantrum. This was not good. He couldn't work out whether it was better than dealing with a panic attack, or worse.

'Kate?' He dropped down beside her and placed a hand on her back. 'What's happened? Talk to me. You're scaring me.'

'Go away,' she said, her voice muffled. 'I don't want you to see me like this.'

'Don't be daft,' he said softly, rubbing her back. 'I'm not leaving you. I need to know you're okay. Can you sit up?'

He wasn't sure she was going to comply, but eventually she rolled onto her back and clumsily sat upright. He almost laughed. Her ponytail was lopsided, she was covered in dead leaves, and her cardigan was stained with mud. At least, he hoped it was mud.

Suki gave her a quick sniff, looked unimpressed and wandered off to explore.

He removed the leaves from her hair. 'Why are you upset?'

Her eyes dropped to her lap. 'I'm fine. I'm just… venting. You don't need to worry about me. I'll get over it.'

'I'm sure you will, but it doesn't mean you're okay right at this moment.' He brushed mud from her sleeve. 'Is it your family? Is someone ill?'

She shook her head. 'Nothing like that.'

'Then what? Because something's wrong.'

Her eyes were still downcast. 'My cousin Beth phoned this morning. She had news about my ex, Tristan.'

'What's the bastard done now? Sold your kidneys on the black market?'

She looked up, startled. For an awful moment, he feared he might have misjudged the situation and she was about to start crying again – or worse, hit him with the discarded branch. But she surprised him by laughing. 'You're right, he is a bastard. A complete and utter selfish arsehole of a bastard.'

'No argument from me.'

But then her smile faded and she started crying again. *Oh, hell.* He reached out to touch her arm and realised her cardigan was damp. She was shaking from the cold as much as from being upset.

He got to his feet and offered her his hand. 'Let's get you to the car, you're freezing.'

She allowed him to pull her upright. 'I have no idea where I am,' she said, gazing around the misty forest. 'I don't even know how I got here.'

'Just as well we found you then.' He steered her towards the path. 'This way.'

She looked disorientated. 'We?'

'Me and Suki.' The dog bounded over when she heard her name but, having deduced there were no treats on offer, wandered off again in disgust.

'Sorry, my brain's a bit fuzzy. I didn't sleep well.'

Deciding she didn't look stable on her feet, he risked sliding an arm around her waist to steady her. She didn't object. In fact, she leant against him, as if content to let him take the lead.

When they reached the car, he called the dog, who gave him a dirty look at having her walk cut short… until he fed her a treat, and just like that he was back in her good books. She was a fickle creature.

Having propped Kate against the car, he fetched a blanket and his spare jacket from the boot. 'Take off your cardigan and put this on,' he said, handing her the puffer jacket.

Her hands were shaking so badly, he had to unclasp the fastening for her. Even her neck was cold. His fingers felt burning hot as they brushed against her skin. She had flecks of mud speckled across her cheeks and he had a strange urge to wipe them away.

Instead, he busied himself shoving the wet cardigan in the boot, waiting until she'd lowered herself into the passenger seat before draping the blanket over her knees.

'How come you have a blanket?' she said, her voice shaky. She looked cute in his jacket.

'I was stuck in a snowstorm a few years back and had to spend the night in my car. It was bloody freezing. After that, I make sure I always have stuff in the boot, in case it happens again. Better?'

'Much better.' She looked up and smiled, and he almost hit his head on the door in his haste to retreat.

He gestured for Suki to jump in the back. The dog wasn't happy about not riding shotgun on the way home, so he pacified her with another treat. Suki must cost Geraldine a fortune in dog treats.

Settling into the driver's seat, he started the engine and turned up the heating. 'You should warm up soon.' He handed her a bottle of water. 'It'll help if you drink something.'

She obediently accepted the bottle and took a swig. 'Sorry about this.'

'That's okay.' He watched her take a deep breath. 'Do you want to talk about it?'

She hesitated. 'Tristan's been working. I know that doesn't sound like a big deal, but he's also been claiming welfare benefits.' She pulled the sleeves of his jacket over her hands. 'He pleaded insolvency to the courts, and told them he was skint and that his girlfriend wasn't earning either, so they couldn't afford to pay anything towards the debts… which is why the bailiffs came after me instead.' Her head dropped against the headrest.

She looked so sad, he desperately wanted to reach across and hold her. Instead, he folded his arms, ensuring he didn't do something he'd later regret.

It was a while before she spoke again. 'A few weeks ago, Beth was on a hen do with some girlfriends in London, when she spotted Tristan working behind the bar at a nightclub. She didn't say anything at the time in case it was a one-off. You know, a bit of cash-in-hand bar work, or something. But just to be sure, she asked the private investigator who works for her to carry out surveillance on him.'

'Your cousin uses a private investigator?'

Kate nodded. 'Mostly to follow cheating husbands prior to a divorce hearing, so the wife can dig up evidence for the courts and prove infidelity.'

'Right.' Calvin raised his eyebrows. 'Cut-throat stuff.'

She gave a shrug. 'Some people go to extraordinary lengths to avoid paying a settlement. Beth objects to that. You don't want to cross her.'

'Duly noted.'

She smiled, but it didn't last long. 'Anyway, the investigator has been following Tristan for the past two weeks and has discovered that not only is he doing bar work, he's also set up another record distribution company and is trading under a false name.'

Calvin frowned. 'So he's not paying his debts because he can't pay them, but because he's deliberately cheating the system?'

'Got it in one.' A tear escaped and trickled down her cheek. 'All this time he's been letting me pay his debts, faking being skint, while he's been earning money and claiming benefits, and taking me for a fool. I feel like such a mug.'

Calvin shifted in his seat. 'Isn't it illegal to falsely claim benefits?'

She nodded. 'He's not only a liar and a cheat, but he's also disrespectful, with no social conscience. He's a snake in the grass, who doesn't even feel guilty or remorseful about what he's done. That's what gets me. There's no shame in the way he's behaved. He doesn't care that he's ruined my life. As long as he's okay, that's all that matters. How can anyone be so… cruel? And to someone they supposedly once loved. I don't get it. I couldn't treat a stranger like that, let alone someone I'd been married to.'

The tears fell more heavily, and Calvin felt around for the packet of tissues he kept in the door console. 'Is there anything you can do about it?' He ripped open the packet.

She freed her hands and took a tissue. 'Report him, you mean? Honestly, I'd rather just clear the last remaining debt and be shot of him for good. I can't bear the idea of dragging this out any longer. If I start disputing the arrangement and they instigate an investigation, it could be months before this mess is resolved. Years even, and I've had enough.'

'Seems unfair that he gets away with it.'

'Who said life was fair?' She wiped her eyes. 'Certainly not me.' Her head dropped against the headrest. 'Sorry, I'm being a right moody cow. You don't need this. I'm just feeling aggrieved, I'll get over it.'

'You've nothing to apologise for.'

She rolled her head to face him. 'Are you kidding me? I've had another meltdown and you just witnessed me beating the crap out of a tree.'

He tried for a smile. 'At least you didn't have a panic attack. That's progress.'

'Right. Instead of hyperventilating, I've switched to committing ABH on plant life.' She rubbed her face. 'Christ, you must be regretting the day you met me.'

He took a quick swig of water. 'Actually, I envy you.'

Her expression turned incredulous. 'How on earth could a man like you… all handsome and talented and amazing, possibly be envious of a pathetic mess like me?'

She thinks I'm amazing? She really wasn't thinking straight.

'Because at least you're letting go of your frustration and anger. You're not bottling it up inside and pretending everything's okay, when it's not.' He rubbed condensation away from the window. 'I'm sorry for how I reacted on Friday night when you tried to talk to me about it. You were right, I'm not okay. And I have no idea how to deal with that.'

A beat passed. 'Well, I don't recommend tree-bashing.'

He couldn't help smiling. 'No? It looked cathartic.'

'It also leaves splinters.' She held out her hand.

He took it and spotted a pine needle digging into her flesh. 'Hold still.'

'*Ouch.*'

'Nearly done.' He soaked a tissue in the bottled water and used it to wipe her cut clean. She had small hands, or maybe they just looked small because of her clipped nails. 'How come you have such short nails?'

'Habit, I guess. I had to keep them short for playing the piano and guitar. It would seem weird to grow them now. My cousin Megan has these really long, fancy gel nails. I've no idea how she manages to do anything with them, I'd be forever poking my eye out.'

He smiled, recalling numerous occasions when Ainsley had broken a nail and dashed off to the nail bar in a panic, as thought she'd broken her leg. God knows how much time and money she'd spent in that place, not that he'd minded. In contrast, Kate's nails were short, neat and clean, no varnish in sight. 'All done.'

'Thanks.'

Strangely, she hadn't removed her hand, and for some reason he hadn't let go either. 'Feeling warmer?'

'Toasty, thanks.'

'I'll ask Geraldine to make you something hot for breakfast when we get back to the care home. Don't even think about arguing with me.'

'Wouldn't dream of it.' Her eyes slid to his and for a moment everything stilled. The air inside the car seemed to grow even warmer, adding to the steam rising up from the windows.

Suki's sudden bark made them both jump. The dog clearly wasn't happy about playing gooseberry.

Calvin let go of Kate's hand and started the engine. 'I guess we'd better get going.'

Kate wrapped her arms around herself. 'Absolutely.'

Silence descended, and for a while neither of them spoke, as they headed towards the care home. But as they passed Pinnock Farm, Kate pointed outside the window. 'They're selling Christmas trees. Can we stop and get one?'

He slowed the car. 'For the care home?'

'We can put it in the lounge. The residents will love it.' She sounded excited, and after the upset of the morning, it seemed like an easy way to cheer her up.

'Sure,' he said, turning into the farm entrance. 'Why not?'

They parked up by a field full of Christmas trees, all different shapes and sizes. A few people were milling around, but it wasn't busy – the weather had probably put most people off.

Leaving a sulking Suki in the back seat, they got out of the car and went over to inspect the pre-cut trees, grouped into height order.

'What about this one?' he said, selecting a four-foot spruce.

'Too small.' She skipped off, checking out the rest of the trees, before eventually pointing to a huge six-foot Nordmann fir. 'The lounge has high ceilings. We need this one.'

He went over. 'Kate, we'd never get a tree that size in my car.'

She grinned at him. 'I know, and that's why it needs to be this one.'

'Excuse me? You've lost me.'

'Well, you've just admitted to me that you're not okay. I'm guessing that's the first time you've properly acknowledged that.' She watched his face. 'Am I right?'

'I guess.' Outwardly, anyway. Internally, he'd known he was messed up for months. 'But I'm still not following you. What on earth has not being okay got to do with choosing a tree that's too big for my car?'

She stepped closer and rested her hands on his chest. 'Admitting there's a problem is the first step on the road to recovery.'

He looked into her light blue eyes. 'Did you hit your head when you fell in the woods?'

She blinked up at him. 'Now, you can either face the problem head-on and find a solution—'

'Are you suffering from hypothermia?' He placed a hand on her forehead. 'A fever?'

'…Or avoid dealing with the issue, in which case the problem never goes away.'

He lowered his hand, perplexed by her reasoning. 'My problems are not going to be solved by the size of the tree we buy.'

She lifted her hands. 'How do you know that?'

'Okay, I'm taking you to A & E.' He caught her hand and dragged her away, ignoring her laughter. 'You need medical assistance. That splinter was obviously infected and you have tetanus.'

Still laughing, she tugged on his hand, pulling him to a stop. 'Think how great you're going to feel when we overcome the challenge of tree versus car, and we arrive back at the home with the most amazing specimen anyone's ever seen. You'll be thanking me for pushing you.'

He turned, causing her to bump into his chest. 'Are you serious?'

'As a heart attack.' And then she gasped. 'Oh, shit. Sorry!' Her hands covered her mouth. 'God, I'm so sorry, Cal.' Her expression was part mortification, part laughter.

He had no idea why, but her calling him *Cal* almost wiped his feet out from under him.

Maybe it was the challenging glint in her eye as she'd said it, daring him on, or the way she was smiling, inviting him into her batshit crazy world of lunacy… but to his utter shock, he opened his mouth and said, 'Fine. The bigger tree it is.'

Chapter Thirteen

Tuesday, 14th December

When the alarm sounded on her phone, Kate couldn't believe it was midday already. No wonder she kept working through her breaks: time flew by when she was engrossed.

Switching off the alarm, she stood up from the desk and stretched, stiff from sitting for so long. Her back was sore from trying to lift and transport a six-foot Norwegian Christmas tree home yesterday, the memory of which made her smile. She wasn't sure which part amused her most: trying to secure the tree to the roof of Calvin's car, watching him drive home while unable to see through the mass of branches flopping onto the windscreen, or the pair of them standing in the lounge, having finally erected the damned thing, soaking wet and covered in pine needles.

Smiling, she closed the lid on her laptop and went in search of Calvin.

Yesterday had certainly been a day of contrasting emotions. One that had seen her fluctuate from the depths of despair to laughing so hard she hadn't been able to breathe. The end result had been utter exhaustion, and she'd collapsed into bed last night and slept better than she had in months. She hadn't even woken when the windows had blown open in the night, so they were still banging about this morning when she'd finally surfaced. Waking up to find the room freezing hadn't been pleasant, but she'd happily trade that for a decent night's sleep.

Walking across the lobby, she stuck her head around the dining room door, surprised to find it empty. There was no one in the kitchen either, which was odd, considering it was lunchtime. Geraldine would normally be in there, singing along to the radio as she prepared lunch. Where was everyone?

In fact, when she stopped to listen, she realised the care home was eerily quiet.

Puzzled, she returned to the library and tentatively knocked on Calvin's door. She wasn't about to make the same mistake as last time and march into his apartment unannounced. The recollection of him stark naked still had the ability to send waves of heat coursing through her. Not that her behaviour since had been much better. Continually making a fool of herself seemed to be her default setting. As yesterday had proved, when once again she'd emotionally imploded, and he'd been there to not only witness it, but also pick up the pieces.

A soft voice called out, 'Come in,' and she slowly eased the door open to peer inside.

If she'd been shocked to discover him naked last time, she was even more thrown to see him slowly pacing the room with Jacob cradled in his arms. The sight did nothing to dampen the heat in her cheeks.

'He's just gone to sleep,' Calvin whispered, his face breaking into one of those kilowatt smiles. 'Everything okay?'

She wasn't sure what rattled her most: the unleashing of his dimples or the sight of him cradling a baby. Her insides squirmed with longing, and she had to forcibly squash her hormones, which had gone into overdrive. Life really wasn't fair sometimes.

'Everything's fine,' she whispered, wanting to move closer, but resisting for the sake of self-preservation. 'Where is everyone? The place is empty.'

'Esme and Rowan have taken a taxi into Ashford to do some Christmas shopping. Geraldine made an early lunch for Deshad and Priya so she could take the afternoon off, and Larry's out for the day with his son, who's visiting from the States.'

'And Hanna?'

'Hanna's asleep upstairs.'

Kate couldn't have been more surprised if he'd said Hanna's favourite colour was blush-pink. 'Really? During the day?' Maybe she really was a vampire.

'She was up all night covering for Natalie. I insisted she get some rest. Natalie's not feeling so great, so she's gone to see the doctor.'

'Ah, which explains why you've been left holding the baby.' Kate risked moving closer, unable to resist taking a peek at a sleeping Jacob. 'Do you mind looking after him?'

'Mind?' He looked surprised. 'Look at him. He's adorable.'

Kate felt her stomach flip. 'You like babies?'

'I love them,' he said, gazing tenderly down at Jacob. 'But it makes me miss my nieces.' He lowered his head and kissed Jacob's forehead. 'I'm in danger of getting broody.'

He wasn't the only one.

And then he looked up and caught her expression. 'What?'

'Nothing… It's just, not many men would openly admit to feeling broody.'

He shrugged. 'I've always known I wanted kids. I don't think that's anything I should feel embarrassed about.'

'Oh, goodness, of course not,' she said, feeling mortified. 'To be honest, I'm a bit sensitive when it comes to the whole baby thing. I'm not used to someone being so honest about their feelings. It's my hang-up, not yours. I apologise.'

He raised an eyebrow. 'Tristan the bastard, again?'

'The one and only. He told me he wanted kids, but he kept finding excuses for us to wait. It was never the right time, or we needed to be more financially stable – one excuse after another. And then when everything came to light about his debts, I also discovered he'd been sleeping with our next-door neighbour and she was pregnant.'

Calvin's eyes grew wide. 'Christ, he really did a number on you, didn't he?'

She nodded. 'It was the lies that hurt the most. It wasn't that he didn't want kids; he just didn't want them with me, and my self-esteem is struggling to recover from that.'

'Understandably.' He watched her for a moment. 'Fancy a cuddle?'

The heat in her cheeks flamed and she instinctively took a step back – until she realised he was talking about Jacob, and she felt like such an idiot. Of course he wouldn't be offering to cuddle her himself. What was she thinking?

'Unless it's too painful?' he said, looking concerned. 'I know sometimes cuddling other people's kids can fill you with so much love you think you're going to burst, and then other times it's just a painful reminder of what you don't have.'

Crikey, he really did get it.

Hot tears pricked her eyes. 'My cousin Megan's pregnant, and although I'm genuinely delighted for her—'

'It feels like someone's ripped your heart out?'

She nodded. 'Got it in one.'

'I get it, believe me.' He offered her the baby, and when she nodded, he gently slid Jacob into her arms. The manoeuvre meant they were so close, she could feel the warmth radiating through his soft blue hoodie, the tickle of his breath as it skimmed her cheek, and the solid weight of his arm grazing her breast. 'Did you need me for something?'

She looked up. 'Sorry?'

His face was inches away from hers, his brown eyes darkened by dilated pupils. 'You were looking for me earlier?'

'Oh, right… yes, I was. I'm taking your advice and having a lunch break. I thought I could make myself useful and decorate the tree.'

With Jacob secure in her arms, she stepped away, needing to dispel the effect Calvin was having on her.

'But I'm not sure whether you have any decorations, or whether I need to buy some.' Not that she could afford to buy decorations, but there might be a pound shop nearby where she could spend a few quid. Her overdraft wasn't going down anytime soon anyway.

'You're not spending your money on decorations for us. Besides, we already have some.' He moved over to a sideboard and pulled it away from the wall, revealing a small door. 'My uncle kept them under here. Are you all right holding Jacob?'

'Of course. He's out for the count.' She gazed down at him sleeping and a rush of something washed over her. It was just as Calvin had described: a disabling mixture of pleasure and pain.

In the past, she'd always felt guilty for feeling sad when a friend or relative announced their good news. Now she realised it was inevitable and, more importantly, totally understandable.

She watched Calvin crawl into the narrow space. 'How many secret rooms do you have here?'

'Loads,' he said, his voice fading as he disappeared inside. 'The place is full of them.'

Kate took advantage of the wait to enjoy savouring the weight of Jacob lying in her arms. *Will I ever experience this?* she wondered. It seemed increasingly unlikely. Time was running away from her. Still, there was nothing she could do about it. Her focus remained on getting herself financially stable and ridding herself of crippling debt.

Calvin reappeared, carrying a box with the word *Christmas* scrawled on the side in his uncle's distinctive handwriting. 'There are two more,' he said, disappearing back inside.

When all three boxes had been retrieved, he stood up and brushed cobwebs away from his hoodie, visibly shuddering. 'Do I have any spiders in my hair?'

'Several.'

Like a lightning bolt, he whipped off his hairband and chucked his head forwards, frantically shaking out his mass of curly hair. 'Have they gone?'

'I'm joking!' Her laughter didn't stop the guilt she felt at seeing his panic. 'I'm sorry, that was mean of me. There're no spiders in your hair, I promise.'

He straightened and gave her a loaded look. 'I suppose you think you're funny?'

She offered him an apologetic smile. 'Sorry. My attempt at humour.'

He scraped his hair into a high ponytail, revealing the freshly shaved section below, and secured it with the band. 'I'll remember that next time you freak out when you think you've seen a ghost.'

'No, you won't.' She smiled at his disgruntlement. 'And I told you, I don't believe in ghosts.'

He stacked the boxes and carried them from the room. 'You sure about that?'

'Positive.' Carefully holding Jacob, she followed him into the library. 'My mental health issues have nothing to do with paranormal activity. I've achieved bonkers status all by myself.'

Laughing, he glanced back. 'You're not bonkers, you're... wounded. There's a difference.'

'It still equates to me embarrassing myself on a regular basis, as you witnessed only yesterday.'

'You didn't embarrass yourself.' He stopped by the door. 'And what did you mean when you said: "No, you won't?" How do you know I won't retaliate?'

It was a moment before she realised what he meant. 'Ah, right. I said that because you're a nicer person than me. Sad, but true.'

His eyes lifted to hers. 'You're nice... when you're not torturing me by telling me I have spiders in my hair.'

She gave him a sheepish grin. 'Sorry about that.'

'I doubt that.' He rolled his eyes and nodded at the door. 'Can you get the door for me?' And then he realised she had her hands full, too. 'Forget I said that.' He used his hip to release the handle and hooked his foot around the door to pull it open.

'Very smoothly done.'

He headed into the lobby. 'Where's Alex today?'

'Gone to get his hair cut. Hanna's comment that he resembled a scarecrow made him self-conscious. I just hope he doesn't come back with a shaved undercut like hers.'

'Or mine?' Calvin glanced back, one eyebrow raised.

'You can get away with it, he can't.'

'Meaning?'

She followed him into the lounge. 'On you it looks trendy and cool. It matches your tattoos and fashionable style. Alex's hair is like mine, limp and painfully Caucasian. We'd end up looking like plucked chickens.'

Calvin laughed. 'I might have to change my appearance if I get a new job. I'm not sure this look would work in an office.' He lowered the boxes to the floor.

'Depends on which office. Having said that, I can't see you working behind a desk.'

He ripped off the tape on the first box. 'No?'

'You'd be better off doing something team-orientated and hands-on. You know, like running a care home.'

He pinned her with a glare. 'Have you been talking to Esme?'

She feigned innocence. 'No, why?'

'Let's just say, she feels the same way.' He removed the tape from the other two boxes and lifted the lids.

'You're very good at it, but I guess that doesn't count for much if you don't enjoy it. Nothing's worse than a job you hate.'

Calvin removed a handful of shiny tinsel. 'You have a choice: continue holding the baby or putting up the decorations?'

'You start and I'll take over,' she said, heading for the sofa. 'I'm not done cuddling, even if he does weigh a ton.' She gazed down at Jacob as she slid onto the sofa. 'He makes a surprisingly good radiator.'

'You should try holding two of them,' he said, emptying the contents of the box onto the floor. 'My nieces climb on top of me at the same time and it's like holding a couple of baked potatoes.'

Kate laughed, mostly at how northern he sounded saying 'baked potatoes'. 'How old are they?'

'They'll be two in January.' He sorted through the decorations, pausing when he came across a piece of brown plastic.

'Are you hoping to see them over Christmas?'

'I doubt that will happen. I can't see me getting home before things are sorted here. But hopefully I'll see them for their birthdays.' He sounded distracted as he searched through the upturned pile of decorations, gathering together bits of plastic.

'What have you found?'

He sat back on his haunches. 'My Pop-Up Pirate game. It's broken.'

She could tell from his expression that he was upset. 'Was it a favourite toy?'

'Yeah, it was.' He inspected the broken plastic. 'It was the last present my dad gave me before he left. I didn't know at the time it was going to be the last present, but I loved it. I played with it for hours, drove my brother and sister mad by insisting we keep playing another round.' He rubbed a temple, as if confused. 'I don't know how it ended up here.'

Jacob made a noise, attracting her attention. His brief wriggle was followed by a yawn and him drifting back to sleep. 'Can it be fixed?'

'Doesn't look like it.' He got up and threw the pieces in the bin. 'Silly, really. It's not like it was an expensive gift or anything special. It's daft to feel upset about it.'

'It's not daft, at all. It's not the toy itself, but the memory it conjures up. It reminds you of your dad, and that's bound to be painful.' As she knew only too well – even though she had no actual memories of her dad, only recounted stories from other family members. She had no treasured gifts or belongings, not even his guitar anymore, thanks to her arsehole of an ex-husband.

Having binned the broken toy, Calvin set about untangling the tree lights.

She felt bad, watching him do everything, so she lifted Jacob onto the sofa and surrounded him with cushions so he wouldn't roll off. 'Do you think he'll be okay like that?'

Calvin glanced over. 'He'll be fine. It's not like we can't keep an eye on him.' Despite this, he took the cushions from the other sofa and placed them on the floor next to the sleeping baby. 'Just in case.'

Happy that Jacob was safe, Kate joined Calvin on the floor and helped him unravel the lights. 'Was the plan to have kids with your girlfriend one day? You know, before you broke up,' she asked, curiosity getting the better of her.

'That was the plan.' He stretched out the wires and unhooked a few more.

'What happened? If you don't mind me asking.'

'I'm still not entirely sure,' he said, untangling the cord. 'How are you getting on at your end?'

'Almost done.' She released the last of the knots and handed him the lights.

He got up and carried them over to the wall socket. 'Hey, they work,' he said, when he plugged them in.

She dragged a chair over to the tree and stood on it. 'Pass them up, then.'

His expression turned wary. 'You don't have a great track record with stepladders.'

'Which is why I'm on a chair,' she said, her exaggerated eye-roll making him laugh.

He came over and handed her the lights. 'I'm not sure the health and safety officer would agree it's any safer.'

She stretched up to hook the lights over the tree. 'Who is the health and safety officer?'

He paused. 'Me, I guess.'

'Well, that's okay then.' She looked down and smiled. 'It's probably easier if you circle the tree with the lights and I'll spread them out.'

'Whatever you say... Hey, careful there,' he said, catching her when she wobbled. 'Are you sure you're okay up there?'

She lifted her hands, demonstrating her balancing skills. 'See? Perfect core stability.'

He raised an eyebrow and began circling the tree with the lights. 'I don't know who to keep a closer eye on, you or Jacob.'

'Harsh. Although to be fair, I do seem to cry a lot more than him.' She spaced out the lights as he draped them around the tree, her thoughts drifting back to their earlier conversation. 'So you didn't see it coming with your girlfriend?'

'Nope,' he said, adjusting the lights. 'I thought we were happy.' And then he paused. 'To be fair, when I look back, I see things I didn't at the time. Does that make sense?'

'Perfect sense. I'm an expert in hindsight analysis.'

'Well, I wish I was,' he said, stripping off his hoodie. 'Christ, I'm hot.'

Kate tried not to stare the flash of bare stomach as his T-shirt rode up. He might not play sport anymore, but his physique didn't seem to have suffered. She swallowed awkwardly. The sight of the muscles flexing in his tattooed forearms was oddly distracting. 'What kinds of things?'

He handed her a bauble. 'Nothing major. For the most part she was a great girlfriend,' he said, watching her stretch up to place the decoration. 'Do you need to move the chair?'

'No, it's fine.' The chair wobbled. 'On second thoughts, you're probably right.'

Resting her hands on his shoulders, she intended to jump down, but he lifted her instead and lowered her slowly to the floor. Finding herself momentarily airborne was rather alarming. Although not as alarming as when her chest connected with his and her body slid down his, until her feet found the floor. There was a long drawn-out moment, when neither of them moved.

Eventually, she found her voice. 'I sense a but coming...?'

He held her gaze a fraction longer, before moving away, leaving a rush of cold air in his wake. 'There were times when she was a little obsessed about her image and how many followers she had on Instagram.' He went in search of more baubles. 'I didn't understand why it mattered, but clearly it did. She'd get annoyed with me for not taking her side, even though I felt I was on her side, and then it was radio silence for a few days. I learnt to ride it out and wait for her to start speaking to me again.' He gave a brief shrug. 'Apart from that, it was good. It only changed when I got my diagnosis.'

After checking that Jacob was okay, Kate resumed hanging baubles. They had an antique quality to them. The images had faded, but she could faintly make out Victorian skaters on a lake, and carollers grouped around a candlelit tree. 'In what way did things change?'

He kicked off his trainers. It was his turn to climb on the chair.

She tried not to stare at his exposed lower back, as his T-shirt lifted when he stretched upwards. Of course he had a perfectly sculpted back. Why was she even surprised?

She pulled her top down over her very untoned bottom.

'At first, she was shocked, like I was. And then she got angry, said she couldn't understand why I wouldn't carry on playing, even though the club refused to allow it. She wanted me to find another club abroad, who weren't bothered about insurance.' He stepped off the chair and repositioned it.

Kate rummaged through the last box, unearthing a few strands of gold ribbon. Struck by an idea, she glanced at Calvin. Dare she? *Oh, what the hell.*

She discreetly reached for his trainers.

'I tried explaining that it didn't matter where I played, the risk of me dropping dead of heart failure wasn't going away,' he said, climbing back onto the chair. 'And then she became prickly and critical, less sympathetic… that's when she started questioning our future together.'

When Kate was sure he was distracted hanging baubles, she removed his shoelaces and replaced them with gold ribbons. 'Is that when she broke things off?'

His short laugh was loaded with sarcasm. 'It might have been easier if she had. Nope, the next thing I knew, she'd hooked up with a teammate of mine.'

Kate blinked up at him. 'Oh, Calvin, that's awful.'

'And just like that, I'd been replaced. She'd upgraded to a wealthier and healthier version.' He rubbed his chin. 'Sorry, that makes me sound callous.'

'Far from it. Crikey, she could give Tristan a run for his money.' She got up and held out her hand. 'Need help getting down?'

At least that brought a smile to his face. 'I can manage, thanks.'

'Sure? Only, I'm stronger than I look.' She placed her hands on his waist, like he'd done with her, and tried to lift him. 'Or, maybe not.'

Laughing, he climbed off the chair. 'Nutter... Ready for the big reveal?'

'Let's do this. Hang on.' She ran over to the main light switch and flicked it off. 'So we get the full effect.'

Calvin switched on the socket and the tree lit up with flashing coloured lights.

'Pretty,' she said, coming over to admire their work. 'It looks almost Dickensian.'

He stood next to her. 'Is that a polite way of saying the decorations are a bit old?'

'No, I love them. They have character. And besides, they're better quality than you can buy in the shops these days.'

They stood like that for a few seconds, mesmerised by the lights and content to enjoy the silence, broken only by the tick of the grandfather clock. It was oddly calming.

Acting on impulse, she slid her hand into his and gave it a squeeze. She had no idea whether it was the right thing to do, but he'd been so kind to her during her numerous meltdowns so it seemed fitting to offer him some comfort in exchange. She imagined it wasn't easy for him to talk about his feelings.

When his fingers closed around hers, she inwardly sighed. She hadn't messed up. 'I'm so sorry, Cal. You really haven't had a great time of it, have you?'

He leant into her a little. 'What a pair we are, eh?'

'We could win a gold medal in who has the shittiest life competition.'

She felt rather than saw him smile. 'Ah, but we did overcome the tree–versus–car battle.'

'This is true. And if I do say so myself, we've done a sterling job decorating this tree.'

'We have indeed.' His hand squeezed tighter, and then he spotted his trainers lying on the floor. 'What the *f*…?'

She tried to look innocent. 'Something the matter?'

He turned to her. 'You think you're funny, don't you?' He caught her around the middle, before she could escape.

'I don't know what you mean,' she said, squealing. 'No, not tickling!' She tried to wriggle free, but he wasn't letting up. 'That's not fair. You're cheating!'

'How am I cheating?' He tipped her backwards, so she was dangling over the sofa. 'You sabotaged my trainers.'

He pulled her upright and she banged against his chest. She found herself looking into his smiling face, and both of them started laughing as she held on to him, loving the way his sadness had completely vanished… until a voice from behind said, 'Wow! That tree looks amazing!'

They instantly jumped apart, like a conjuror's trick, slicing his assistant in two.

'Thanks so much for looking after Jacob,' Natalie said, heading over to the sofa, oblivious to the heated atmosphere. 'How's he been?'

'No problem at all.' Calvin glanced at Kate and then looked away, his expression indicating that he felt as embarrassed as she did. 'Feeling any better?'

'A bit, thanks. Turns out I'm anaemic. The doctor's given me some iron tablets. He said I should feel better soon.' She picked up Jacob from the sofa and cuddled him. 'I'll take him upstairs for a lie-down. Thanks again for looking after him.'

'Sure, no problem.' Calvin picked up the empty boxes. 'I'd better get rid of these.'

'And I'd better get back to work,' Kate said, her swift exit from the room failing to conceal her flustered state.

Quite why she was feeling so hot and bothered, she wasn't sure.

It wasn't like she had feelings for Calvin.

They were just friends... weren't they?

Chapter Fourteen

Thursday, 16ᵗʰ December

When Calvin received a call from the agency, saying they'd managed to find a locum nurse, his first reaction had been relief. He'd had no idea there was a shortage of care providers in the UK – something the agency manager had been quick to point out when he'd queried why it was taking so long. They were competing against other care homes and domiciliary providers, all looking for staff, so there had been no guarantee of finding someone any time soon.

Therefore, getting a call announcing that they had someone who might be willing to provide cover felt like a miracle. It was only as the day wore on that he'd started to worry whether this person would find Rose Court a desirable place to work. They weren't exactly a high-end organisation; they were the corner-shop equivalent of care homes. Something that had become blatantly apparent when he'd met with the national care-home representative last week. If he hadn't known beforehand what they'd been lacking, he certainly did know now.

It had been a quiet couple of days, thankfully free of dramas to contend with. Kate and Alex had been buried away in the library, finalising the accounts for submission to the tax office, and this morning Kate had broken the good news that she'd been able to submit the probate application.

Outwardly, he'd smiled and shared her joy at having met such a momentous milestone. Internally, a horrible sinking feeling had settled over him. Her time working at the care home would soon be drawing to a conclusion, and for some reason that depressed him. Obtaining probate was the answer to all their prayers. Kate could clear her debts and move on with her life, finally free from her pathetic excuse of an ex-husband, and he could rid himself of the care home's responsibilities and return to his old life in Leeds. It should be a time of celebration. So why didn't it feel like a win?

Headlights flashed across the front windows, indicating that the locum had arrived.

Calvin made his way to the front door to greet them. It was another foggy evening, and his long-sleeved T-shirt wasn't enough to keep the chill at bay as he stood on the steps of the care home, waiting.

A young Black guy climbed out of the taxi and hoisted a rucksack onto his shoulder. Having paid the driver, he looked up at the building, no doubt wondering what he'd let himself in for.

Calvin met him halfway and held out his hand. 'I'm guessing you're from the care agency?'

'You guessed right.' He shook Calvin's hand. 'Nelson Amoah.'

'Good to meet you. I'm Calvin. Welcome to The Rose Court Care Home.'

The guy had a strange look on his face. 'As in... Calvin Johnson? The footballer?'

Calvin's stomach dipped. '*Ex*-footballer, but yes, that's me.'

'Oh, my days.' He let out a long whistle. 'What are you doing here, man?'

'It's a long story.' Calvin nodded towards the door. 'Let's head inside, it's cold.'

Nelson followed him up the steps. 'I'm a big fan of yours, man. You sure had some skills on the football pitch.'

Calvin glanced back. 'Thanks.'

'Sorry to hear about your retirement. That was a blow. Gutted for you.'

The guy knew his football. 'I appreciate it.'

'How you doing? You coping okay?'

Calvin almost smiled; this guy would get on well with Kate. 'I'm getting there.' He pointed to the coat stand. 'Leave your coat and rucksack down here, while I show you around, save you carrying everything with you.'

He handed Calvin his bag and removed his coat. He was wearing smart black trousers and a blue nurse's tunic. He certainly looked the part. 'The agency said you don't have many residents?'

'Not at the moment. The care home was run by my late uncle until his death a few months ago. Old age and illness meant a lot of things have slipped over the years, and the place has suffered from a lack of management and money. We're in the process of sorting out the estate so we can make the necessary improvements, but I'll be honest with you, things are still haphazard at the moment.'

Nelson lifted his hands. 'Hey, man. I worked out of a tent in Haiti, following a hurricane; this place is like Buckingham Palace compared to that.'

'You've worked abroad?'

'A few places. Looking for some stability now. Find a girl, start a family. You know the drill.'

Calvin smiled. 'Good luck with that.' He opened the lounge door. 'Come and meet the residents.'

The scene that greeted them when they entered the lounge was a familiar one. The Christmas tree lights were flashing away, the tables were covered in wine bottles, half-drained glasses and bowls of crisps, and the open fire crackled away, throwing off waves of heat. Esme and Rowan were sitting on one sofa, Larry and Deshad on the other.

Geraldine was lying on the floor, frowning at the TV remote. All of them were wearing Christmas jumpers and cracker hats, and had matching rosy cheeks – hence the wine bottles. Considering it was only eight o'clock, they were rattling through the booze.

Esme was the first to notice that their little soiree had been interrupted and waved her hand. 'Ah, the cavalry! Calvin will know how to work the remote, he's very technically minded.'

All heads turned in their direction and the noise level increased, as they broke into simultaneous conversation.

Calvin glanced at Nelson, wondering what the poor guy made of this rather raucous gathering. He couldn't imagine other care homes allowed such boozy evenings. 'Sorry about this. It's movie night. It's not normally so rowdy.'

Nelson grinned. 'It's good to see everyone having fun.'

He was tactful, Calvin would give him that.

'And who do we have here?' Rowan looked far too hot in his bright red 'Santa's Little Helper' jumper.

'This is Nelson, our new locum nurse. I'm giving him the guided tour. Esme, Rowan, Larry and Deshad are all residents here,' he said, gesturing to each one as he introduced them. 'Geraldine over there is our chef... And this is Suki, Geraldine's dog.' Suki trotted over and sniffed Nelson's crotch.

Calvin snapped his fingers, calling the dog away. Embarrassing animal.

'Not that she behaves like she's my dog anymore,' Geraldine said, squinting at the remote. 'She's switched allegiance.' She banged the gadget on the floor. 'What is wrong with this darned thing? Why won't it work?'

Calvin went over. 'What are you trying to do?'

'We want to watch *Scrooge*, but the video won't work.'

Calvin pressed the play button, and when Albert Finney's face appeared on the screen, they all cheered and broke into a round of applause like he'd brokered world peace.

'He's so clever,' Esme said, her elbow slipping off the armrest.

Rowan nodded. 'Youngsters these days are so IT savvy. I don't understand half of what they know.'

'Speak for yourselves,' Geraldine said, sounding grumpy. 'My brain works just fine, thank you. The remote was playing up.'

Rowan blew her a kiss. 'Whatever you say, darling.' He turned to Nelson, his paper hat obscuring one eye. 'You're welcome to join us, young man. We don't stand on ceremony here, the staff let their hair down as much as the residents.'

Calvin inwardly cringed; it hardly made them sound very professional.

'Maybe later,' Nelson said, tactfully. 'Enjoy the film, it's my nanna's favourite.'

Rowan looked delighted. 'Ursula's too.'

Nelson looked around the room. 'Who's Ursula?'

'Oh, Ursula is—'

'A former resident,' Calvin cut in, before they freaked the man out completely. 'We'd better get on with the tour. It's getting late and Nelson needs to settle in.' He ushered Nelson from the room before Rowan could launch himself into one of his ghost stories. 'I'll show you the dining room.'

'Bye, Nelson!' Esme's elbow slipped off the armrest again, spilling wine everywhere.

Rowan waved manically, dislodging his hat completely. 'Lovely meeting you!'

Lucky Larry caught Nelson's eye. 'I bet your training didn't prepare you for this?'

Nelson laughed. 'I'm one of six siblings. This is nothing compared to the Christmases at our house.'

Once in the safety of the lobby, Calvin offered him an apologetic smile. 'Sorry about that. Things aren't normally so unruly.'

'It's Christmas,' he said, with a good-natured shrug. 'They're having fun.'

'The dining room is over here.' Calvin showed him the long room, set up for breakfast. 'And through the back is the kitchen.'

Nelson nodded his approval, admiring the stag antlers on the walls and the open brick fireplace. 'The building has character.'

'It's also falling apart, but we try to focus on the positives. The staff and residents' rooms are upstairs,' he said, heading for the stairwell. 'I mentioned to the agency that free board and lodging are available, if you want to stay over rather than travel here for each shift. Did they pass on that information?'

'Why else d'you think I'm here?' Nelson said, matter-of-factly. 'It means I can send money home to my family in Ghana.'

Fair enough. Calvin was glad he'd thought of adding that detail to the advert. Anything to make the job more appealing. 'The code for the doors is the same on each floor. We don't have any residents with severe dementia at the moment, but for security reasons, we like to keep each floor secure.'

'Makes sense.' Nelson followed him upstairs. 'You still involved in football?'

'Not at the moment.' Calvin noticed dust along the handrail and discreetly wiped it away.

'Shame. It's a loss to the game.'

Calvin opened the door to the first floor, hit by another wave of grief. Would it ever not hurt? He guessed not. 'Do you play?'

'Sunday league. Not quite jumpers for goalposts, but nothing like your level.'

'I no longer have a level.' He closed the door behind them. 'This way.'

'You thought about getting involved in coaching?'

'It's something I might look into. I'm not sure I have the right attributes.'

'We're looking for a coach at our club, if you're interested. We're based in Ashford. The Under 13s would benefit from someone with your football experience.'

Calvin straightened a wonky picture on the wall. 'Thanks for the offer, but I'm not planning on staying in the area. I'll be heading back to Leeds once this place is sorted.'

'Shame. It's hard getting a PAN team off the ground. No one involved in the club has the right skills to adapt the training.'

Calvin stopped walking. 'What's a PAN team?'

'Integrating disabilities. Adult football is divided up by disability, whether it's visual impairment, hearing loss or wheelchair users. But with kids' football, they play according to age band, regardless of their disability. It's a new thing for our club. We haven't had sufficient interest before, but we've got enough kids now to form a team. What we haven't got is a coach who knows enough about football to adapt the training to meet their individual needs.'

Calvin shoved his hands in his jeans pockets. 'I'm not sure I'd be much help. I know nothing about coaching kids with disabilities.'

'But you know what it's like to feel frustrated by your limitations. They want to do everything the other kids do, but they can't. They get upset when they can't run as fast, move as quickly or react to the ball changing direction. They need someone who knows the disappointment of wanting to do more than their body will allow. They love football, but at the moment they don't love playing it, and that's a shame. I thought you might relate to that.'

It was a moment before Calvin could speak. A lump had wedged itself in his throat, preventing him from swallowing. 'Is there an established league for them to play in?'

'Yeah, quite a big one. It covers most of Kent, but it's hard getting a new team off the ground. We train Tuesday evenings, if you fancy coming down.'

'Like I said, I'm not going to be here much longer.' He turned to walk off, hesitated and then turned back. 'But I'll pop down if I can.' He wasn't sure why he'd said that – curiosity, probably. Guilt, more likely. He knew he should give something back to the beautiful game that had given him so much over the years, but he just didn't know how to do that without exacerbating his own suffering.

Nelson's face broke into a smile. 'The kids would love that. A proper star. You'll make their year.'

'No promises. My time's pretty occupied with this place.'

'Fair enough.' Nelson followed him down the corridor. 'So what's the deal here? How many staff do you have on the books?'

'Three. Geraldine, our chef, who you just met, and two full-time nurses. Hanna, who works days, and Natalie, who works nights.'

'That's it?'

Calvin glanced back. 'That's it.'

'No wonder you need a locum.'

'I look after the management side of things, and we have a solicitor and an accountant working for us at the moment who're trying to sort out my uncle's estate. The aim is to free up enough funds to get the business functioning properly, but until that happens, we're running on reduced staffing levels.'

Nelson didn't comment; he didn't have to. Calvin was aware of how dire things were.

They reached the staff room and Calvin could hear bizarre noises coming from inside. For a second, he almost avoided going in there, unsure of what he was about to find, but it would seem even odder to ignore it.

Nothing could have prepared him for the sight of Alex lying prone on the floor, with Hanna kneeling over him, her hands locked together and pressing on his chest. 'Like this…' she said, pretending to pump. '…two… three… four…'

Calvin cleared his throat. 'Sorry to interrupt, guys.'

Hanna looked up, unimpressed. 'Yes?'

'Is Alex okay down there?'

'He fine,' she said, answering for him and sitting back on her haunches. 'I teach him CPR. Everyone should know technique.' Her eyes narrowed. 'You know technique?'

'I do, yes,' he said, fearful of being made to join in the lesson. 'Hanna, this is Nelson, our new locum nurse.'

She got to her feet and marched over. 'Hanna Wozniak, head nurse. You start tonight?'

Nelson shook her hand, buckling under the strength of her grip. 'Tomorrow.'

Hanna frowned. 'Why not tonight?'

'Nelson needs to get accustomed to the place before being expected to start a shift,' Calvin said, willing her to make a good impression so the bloke wouldn't change his mind. They needed him.

'We small team.' She gave him the once-over, taking in his shaved head and tattooed forearms – which was ironic, seeing as how her blue-black hair and multiple piercings were hardly the stereotypical look for a care worker. 'We dedicated to residents. Not afraid of hard work. We *committed*.' Her hands went to her hips. 'You same?'

'Me same,' he said, with a good-natured smile. Calvin almost laughed. 'I think loyalty's important. I'm looking forward to working with you.'

Hanna harrumphed. 'We see.'

Alex got up from the floor. 'Hi, I'm Alex.'

Calvin noticed that the young man's T-shirt was on inside out. 'Alex is the accountant I was telling you about.'

Nelson fist-bumped Alex. 'Good to meet you, man.'

'You too.' Alex ran a hand through his shorter hairstyle, sitting neatly above his collar.

Calvin gestured to the door. 'We'll leave you to get on with your CPR lesson.'

'Eight sharp in morning!' Hanna called out, as they exited. 'No late!'

Nelson glanced back and saluted. 'No late.'

Hanna turned and barked at Alex, 'Back on floor.'

Poor Alex. But instead of obeying, he pinned her with a glare, and said, 'No, Hanna, *you* get on the floor. It's my turn to practise.' He sounded uncharacteristically assertive, causing Calvin to do a double take.

Hanna drew in a sharp breath.

Oh, hell.

A heated pause followed, and Calvin waited for the fallout, but instead of exploding, Hanna rolled her eyes and said, 'Fine,' and dutifully laid down on the floor.

Bloody hell. *Go, Alex*.

'Her bark's worse than her bite,' Calvin said to Nelson, when they were safely out of earshot. 'She's an excellent nurse. You just need to get used to her.'

Nelson grinned. 'I've dealt with worse.'

'You have?'

Nelson laughed. 'I have four sisters.'

They continued down the corridor and came across Natalie. She was seated at the nurses' station, breastfeeding Jacob. It was a common enough sight for Calvin, and he liked to think it made them look progressive as an employer, encouraging inclusivity and equality, but he couldn't imagine it was routine in most workplaces. Would this be the moment their new locum made a run for it?

'This is Natalie, our night nurse.' Calvin braced himself for weirdness, but Nelson didn't bat an eyelid.

'Hi, Natalie. I'm Nelson.' He kept his eyes on her face. 'I'm looking forward to working with you.'

'It's really lovely to meet you. We're so pleased you're here.' Jacob made a gurgling noise. 'And this is my son, Jacob. Apologies in advance if he wakes you in the night with his crying. He's teething.'

Nelson smiled. 'No worries.'

Calvin breathed a sigh of relief. Another hurdle overcome. 'I notice Deshad was in the lounge watching the Christmas film with the others,' he said to Natalie. 'How did you manage to persuade him to take a break?'

'I didn't, Kate did. She offered to sit with Priya for the evening, so he could watch the film. She's in there with her now.'

An odd feeling washed over him and his eyes slid to Priya's door. 'Kate's the solicitor I was telling you about, who's dealing with my uncle's estate.'

'Nice of her to help out.' Nelson sounded part-impressed, part-bemused.

Calvin knew the feeling.

'It is,' he said, turning back. 'Deshad is Priya's husband and main carer. He lives here with her. It's an unusual arrangement, I know.'

Nelson remained unfazed. Nothing rattled him, it seemed. 'Nice they can stay together. More homes should offer that.'

Nelson was turning out to be the perfect fit. Either that, or he was a bloody good actor. Calvin hoped it wasn't the latter.

'Are you okay chatting to Natalie for a moment? I want to stick my head around the door and say hi. I'll introduce you properly tomorrow, but I feel it would be better if Deshad was here when you meet Priya. He's a bit protective of who gets involved in her care.'

'You take your time, man.'

'Thanks.' Calvin left them talking and knocked quietly on Priya's door, before easing it open.

Kate was lying on the bed next to Priya, her laptop open in front of them. She was wearing Christmas pyjamas covered in red-nosed reindeers and her hair was loose. She looked so adorably cute that for a moment he couldn't speak.

'Hi,' she said, looking up. 'We're watching *It's a Wonderful Life*. It's Priya's favourite Christmas movie.'

'I see you're dressed for the part,' he said, coming over to the bed. 'Is it any good?'

'Haven't you seen it?' She patted Priya's hand. 'Did you hear that, Priya? Calvin's never seen the film. He's missing out, isn't he?'

Priya gave a faint nod, making the bells on her elf hat tinkle, but her gaze remained fixed on the laptop screen.

It was then that he noticed Kate's slippers. 'What on earth have you got on your feet?'

'Snowmen.' She wiggled her toes. 'Alex got them for me when he went into town to get his hair cut. Cool, aren't they?'

'Aren't they're supposed to be warm?'

She laughed. 'Are you trying to be funny?'

178

'And failing, clearly.' He smiled, needing a moment to gather his thoughts. She looked so pretty, with her flushed cheeks and messy hair. 'Thanks for doing this,' he said, coming around to her side of the bed. 'It's really kind of you. And it's great to see Deshad joining in with the others for once.'

'It's no big deal,' she said, offering him a bowl of chocolates. 'I'm happy to help. How's your evening going? Has the locum shown up yet?'

'He's outside, talking to Natalie.' He accepted a chocolate. 'His name's Nelson. He seems like a nice guy.'

'Well, that's a relief,' she said, unwrapping a chocolate. 'Why do I sense a but coming?'

He perched on the arm of the chair next to the bed. 'I never realised quite how unconventional this place is until I began showing him around.'

She smiled. 'Personally, I'm in favour of anything unconventional. It makes me feel less insane.' She popped the chocolate in her mouth. 'You think he's going to do a runner?'

'I would, if I were him.' He unwrapped his chocolate.

'And yet you didn't.' She smiled at him. 'Despite everything, you stayed.'

Their eyes met and he felt something warm trickle through him. 'I can't stay forever, though.'

'Neither of us can.' She looked momentarily sad. 'Maybe we just have to view this as an interim step in our lives, a stepping stone we both needed to take to be able to find a new direction in life.'

A weight settled in his chest. 'Maybe.'

'You're not looking very Christmassy,' she said, glancing down at his feet. 'I see you've removed the gold ribbons, spoilsport. I feel quite aggrieved, sat here in festive pyjamas while you're looking all trendy and serious. At least put on a pair of antlers.'

He grinned. 'Not happening.' He ate his chocolate and was hit by a burst of alcohol. 'Christ, what's in these chocolates?'

'Cointreau.' She reached for another. 'Not a fan?'

'You could get drunk on these.' He blinked back tears. 'My eyes are watering.'

She reached for his hand. 'Ah, don't cry. It'll be over soon.'

He laughed. 'Nutter.'

Deciding it was time to leave, before he did something crazy – like settle down and watch the film with her, so he could hold her hand – he got up. Nelson was waiting, and despite feeling reluctant to walk away from Kate in her cute festive outfit, which gave him an uncontrollable urge to snuggle, he couldn't give in to those feelings. That would be bad. For both of them.

'Night-night, Katiekins.' He squeezed her snowman slipper as he passed the end of the bed. 'Night, Priya. Enjoy your film.'

'We will, won't we, Priya?'

He walked away, still puzzled by his feelings.

'Cal…?' When he turned back, she threw a chocolate at him. 'Live dangerously,' she said, with a wink. 'You know you want to.'

He grinned, despite himself.

He would never have thought that Kate Lawrence was his type, but he'd be lying if he said he didn't feel better when she was around. Less morose and more like his old self. The idea that fairly soon they'd be living at opposite ends of the country, with absolutely no reason to be involved in each other's lives, depressed the hell out of him.

Maybe it was just loneliness. He was missing his mates. Ainsley. His family. Kate was easy to be around – she was fun, entertaining and easy to talk to. Becoming attached was inevitable. It didn't mean there was anything significant between them. Like she said herself, they were an interim solution to a bigger problem that needed solving.

He headed into the corridor and closed the door behind him, pleased to see Nelson and Natalie chatting away. He could always rely on her to make a good impression.

'Natalie's been telling me about the residents,' Nelson said, grinning as he leant against the wall. 'They sound like an eccentric group.'

Calvin rolled his eyes. 'That's one word for them.'

'I'm looking forward to getting to know them.'

Calvin paused. 'You mean, you're staying?'

Nelson raised an eyebrow. 'Any reason why I shouldn't?'

'Of course not, it's just… I was worried you might be put off by our quirks.'

'I like quirks.' He pushed away from the wall. 'Where am I sleeping?'

Calvin let out a long breath.

He'd never felt so relieved in his life.

Chapter Fifteen

Sunday, 19th December

For the first time since arriving in Pluckley, Kate was able to enjoy a whole day off. She'd spent the last week finalising the probate forms, ready to send off to the tax office, and she'd entered the final asset into her spreadsheet yesterday. It had taken a month to collate all the information regarding Bert Williams's estate, but it was finally done. The hard work had paid off.

In celebration, she'd gone for a long walk in the morning and rewarded herself afterwards with a hot bath, followed by two large helpings of Geraldine's home-made leek and potato soup. She'd even managed to tinker on the piano while the others had been at church. The place wasn't often empty, and with Hanna safely upstairs tending to Priya, she'd been able to grab an undisturbed twenty minutes before anyone returned.

Pampering herself and getting to play music had felt good, and somehow eased the strange ache that had settled in her chest. She supposed feeling emotional was inevitable. She was exhausted, and hearing the news about Tristan's latest betrayal was bound to sting, but it was the thought of leaving Pluckley that saddened her most. Strangely, Rose Court had begun to feel like home, even with its weird noises and propensity for opening windows in the middle of the night.

Most of all, she was going to miss Calvin. She'd become accustomed to hanging out with him. She wasn't foolish enough to believe anything romantic could happen between them, but she liked to think they'd become friends. He was one of the few people in her life she could truly trust, and she was going to miss that.

The alarm sounded on her phone and she rolled off the bed, placing her bookmark between the pages of her romance saga. It was time to get ready for this evening's Winter Glow event at one of the local mansion houses in the village, Greystones Manor. The temperature had dropped another few degrees, so she layered herself up with warm clothing, picked up her coat and the hat she'd customised, and made her way downstairs to join the others.

When she reached the lobby, she found Geraldine, Esme and Lucky Larry waiting. Esme was looking very chic in a long red coat, and Larry looked like a cool Father Christmas in his green velvet Santa hat.

'Here you are! We were just coming to find you,' Geraldine said, looking hilarious in her Christmas-pudding bonnet. 'Ready to go?'

'Absolutely.' Kate looked around the empty lobby. 'Where's everyone else?'

'Calvin went ahead with Rowan, so he can get ready for his performance, and Hanna and Alex are in the staff room, working on next week's quiz questions.'

'Is that what they're calling it these days?' Esme said, making Larry laugh.

Kate had no idea what they found so amusing, but they were obviously enjoying an in-joke. 'I assume Nelson's looking after Deshad and Priya?' Natalie had gone away for a few days, her first weekend off in months.

'He is, and doing a sterling job.' Esme opened the front door. 'Which just leaves us. The taxi's outside – shall we head off?'

They exited the building and made their way over to the car. Geraldine climbed in the front seat, and Esme and Larry got in the back, which left Kate squashed against the door, her knee digging into the handle.

'Calvin said he'd meet you at the venue,' Esme said, smelling of expensive perfume and a hint of brandy. 'Rowan was keen to get there early, so he could "focus on his craft". He does take these performances rather seriously.'

Kate smiled. 'It's nice he has a hobby. When my grandpa went into a home, he just sat there all day, looking miserable and refusing to join in with any of the activities. At least Rowan's passionate about something, even if it is scaring everyone with his ghost stories.'

Esme laughed. 'They are rather far-fetched, but I agree it's better than sitting around, waiting to die. I can think of nothing worse.'

The taxi pulled away and they began the short drive into the village. 'Fairytale of New York' played on the car radio, accompanied by Geraldine and Larry singing along.

Esme dipped her head closer to Kate. 'Calvin tells me you had a similar upbringing to his. Did he mention his father left when he was young?'

Kate drew back, feeling awkward at the direct line of questioning. 'Er... yes, he did.'

'I suspected as much. Apart from making my daughter's life hell, it had rather a negative impact on Calvin. He never cried, you know. But it did change him. My beautiful, smiling, happy grandson became very quiet and withdrawn. He took it upon himself to become the father figure of the family and look after his younger siblings.'

Kate shifted position. 'It doesn't surprise me. He's certainly taken on the responsibility when it comes to dealing with his uncle's estate.'

'And that's my concern,' Esme said, keeping her voice low. 'He has a habit of sacrificing himself for others. He has a strong sense of duty, and I'm worried he's slipped into another period of acute sadness, for want of a better description. When it happened before, he had football to focus on. But without that in his life, I worry for his mental health.'

Kate wished the driver would put his foot down. Talk about an uncomfortable conversation. 'Why are you telling me this?'

'I want you to understand that Calvin isn't as confident as he appears.'

'Well, I think that's evident.'

'Is it?' Esme seemed surprised. 'Only, Ainsley never understood that about him. She never really saw Calvin the man, only Calvin the successful footballer. It meant their relationship was rather… how can I put this? Superficial. From her side of things, anyway.' She rested her hand over Kate's. 'He finds it difficult to open up and admit to his inner struggles. But I sense he's more comfortable talking to you than anyone else, and I wanted to say that whatever you're doing, thank you, because it's working. You have no idea how wonderful it is to see him smiling again.'

'I'm just being a friend,' she said, feeling increasingly awkward. 'And he's helped me a lot more than I've helped him.'

Esme squeezed her hand. 'You're helping each other, and it's lovely to see.'

Thankfully, the taxi pulled up at their destination, ending the conversation. Kate wasn't comfortable talking about Calvin in this way – it felt too intrusive, like she was betraying his trust, and that didn't sit right. But it did confirm one thing: she couldn't subject him to any more of her meltdowns. It wasn't fair on him; he had his own demons, and dealing with her instabilities couldn't be doing him any good. From now on, she would keep her issues under wraps and enjoy spending her last few days with him.

Calvin must have been watching out for their arrival, because he jogged over to the taxi and helped them out. He looked his usual trendy self: designer jacket over a warm hoodie, his jeans faded and ripped at the knees.

She unearthed his baseball hat from her pocket. 'You'll need this, it's freezing.'

'I've been looking for that all day,' he said, taking it from her. 'Where did you find it?'

She tried not to look guilty. 'I may have pinched it.'

'What do you mean, you may have pinched it?'

'I felt you needed to get into the Christmas spirit more. Don't worry, it's nothing permanent. Just a minor adjustment.'

Unfolding his hat, he stared in disbelief at the cartoon reindeer loosely stitched to the front. 'I'm not wearing this,' he said, sounding appalled. 'I'll look a right idiot.'

'Oh, please.' She placed her Christmas-tree hat on her head and switched on the battery-operated lights. 'Next to me you'll look positively normal.'

His expression switched to a grin. 'I am not walking around with you wearing that.'

'Sure you are.' She took the baseball cap from him and reached up to place it on his head. It meant her chest bumped against his, but thankfully several layers of clothing deadened the impact of touching him. 'There. You fit in now.'

When he looked down at her, she was hit by how much she was going to miss seeing his dimpled smile every day.

'Sorry I stole your hat,' she said, smiling at the sight of him wearing it.

'You're forgiven. At least it'll shut Rowan up. He saw me searching for it and told Nelson that Ursula had taken it.'

'How did Nelson take the news of Ursula?'

'Surprisingly calmly. Apparently, in Ghana a spirit living in your home is considered good luck.'

'And to think you were worried he might not fit in.'

Calvin shook his head. 'Who knew, right?'

A bell rang and everyone started moving towards the house. A thin coating of ice had formed across the tarmac, making walking slightly precarious.

Calvin must have noticed her struggle, because he caught her elbow. 'I still can't get over that hat. Did you make it?'

They reached the safety of the gate and she was able to move onto safer ground. 'Rowan gave me the hat and I added the lights.'

'I suppose I should be grateful you didn't add lights to mine.'

'Oh, I considered it,' she said, smiling. 'But even I knew that was a step too far.'

'Good decision.'

'But we'll have you in a full Santa outfit by Christmas Day.'

He laughed. 'Not going to happen.'

The crowd moved to the back of the house, where thankfully the ground was less slippery.

Greystones was a huge grey building, with a multitude of windows and an imposing air.

'It looks like a very serious house,' she said, gazing up at the mass of icicle lights decorating the rooftop. 'I already know something bad happened here. You can feel it.'

'Like being made to wear a reindeer hat?'

'And I thought Rowan was dramatic?'

'Talking of Rowan.'

She looked over to where he was pointing. 'Oh, good God. I'm guessing he's not trying to be funny?'

'Who knows.'

Rowan was dressed as a monk. He wore long brown robes, tied around the middle with thick rope that swung around his legs as he walked.

'His feet must be freezing,' she said, spotting his open-toed sandals. 'But it's the wig that steals the show.' He was wearing a bald cap, with a band of hair running from ear to ear.

'And I thought nothing could top the ridiculousness of *your* hat,' Calvin said, nudging her.

She feigned offence. 'My hat is tasteful. And fun. And very festive.'

'And very bonkers,' he said, smiling, when she poked her tongue out at him.

The grounds surrounding Greystones couldn't really be called a garden. There was no boundary or fencing, just an expanse of lawn merging seamlessly into the woodland leading down to a lake. The area nearest the house had been landscaped, with rustic steps leading down to a seating section. The borders were lit by solar-powered flowers that formed an impressive light display.

'No wonder there're so many visitors, it's beautiful,' she said, watching the lights shoot up from the centre of the water fountain.

'I thought you'd like it.'

She turned to him. 'Have you been here before?'

'We spent a few Christmases here when I was younger. My uncle would always bring us to the light show.'

'Maybe that's how your Pop-Up Pirate game ended up at the care home... you brought it with you when you came to visit once?'

He seemed surprised. 'You have a good memory.'

She shrugged. 'It clearly meant a lot to you.'

A gong sounded, drawing their attention to the patio area. A man dressed in Dickensian attire addressed the crowd. 'Ladies and gentlemen! Welcome to our annual Christmas light-show event!'

Everyone cheered.

'We shall begin this evening's entertainment with the tale of a local legend. Please welcome to the stage, renowned historian, Rowan Blakely.'

Rowan swept onto the patio, his arms aloft – and almost went flying headfirst when he trod on the bottom of his robes.

Calvin stifled a laugh.

Rowan launched into his monologue. 'Aside from the architectural splendour you see before you, Greystones Manor carries with it the pain and suffering of a former resident, a monk who drifts amongst the surrounding grounds and trees in mournful solitude. He is said to have lived in Tudor times, and is reputed to have fallen in love with the mistress of a neighbouring property.'

Rowan gestured to a woman wearing a fancy period gown. 'But the lady died under tragic circumstances, and following her death, he sank into a state of melancholy. His only solace was to walk the green fields and leafy lanes where they had enjoyed so many romantic interludes together.'

He blew the woman a kiss.

When Calvin stifled another laugh, Kate nudged him. 'Behave.'

Rowan held his hand dramatically against his forehead. 'But as time passed, he sank deeper into depression, pining for his dead lover, and finally died of a broken heart. His ghost continues to wander the neighbourhood, drifting behind the house, in search of his lost love.'

It took the crowd a moment to realise he'd finished, so the clapping came in bursts, before everyone joined in.

'He should win an Oscar,' Calvin whispered in Kate's ear.

'He's enjoying himself, and that's all that matters.'

'You sound like my gran after I was forced to play a wise man in the school nativity. "At least you enjoyed yourself, love." If I hadn't known I sucked beforehand, I did afterwards.'

Kate couldn't help laughing. It was hard to imagine Calvin performing in a school play. 'Is that where your aversion to dressing up comes from?'

'No, that comes from being of sound mind.'

She stemmed her laughter when the woman dressed in Tudor clothes stepped forwards to begin her performance. 'Ladies and gentlemen, if you look towards the skyline, you will see the turret of Rose Court in the distance, a large house situated on the Pluckley Road. It has stood for hundreds of years and is thought to have been built as a home for the mistress of a son of Lord Dering, and it is this lady's ghost which to this day haunts the house.'

Kate's eyes grew wide. 'Is she talking about Ursula?'

Calvin nodded. 'The one and only.'

Kate's attention immediately reverted to the woman.

'The story goes that she fell in love with a monk who lived here at Greystones and found the love triangle so distressing that she took her own life by drinking the juices of poisonous

189

berries. The reason for her suicide remains unconfirmed, but if all that has been said is true, then an emotional entanglement could well have been the cause. To be a Dering mistress and at the same time enjoy a relationship with another man may have created a pressure too great to bear.'

Kate inwardly flinched, as she always did with any mention of suicide. It didn't matter that it was a fanciful legend from centuries past, the idea that anyone could be so heartbroken as to end their life saddened her. It wasn't hard to fathom why.

The woman continued. 'From the position of her body, it would seem that her final moments were spent gazing across the fields in the direction of Greystones, the home of her lover.'

Calvin's arm slipped around Kate, and she leant into him, glad of the comfort.

'Over the years, the residents of Rose Court have reported a number of strange occurrences. Articles that mysteriously move, windows opening in the dead of night and the sound of strange groaning echoing through the rooms in the early hours. A peculiar eerie atmosphere hangs over the house, and to this day the Tudor Lady remains restless, searching for resolution and peace.'

The woman took a bow and the crowd applauded. Rowan joined her on the makeshift stage and they took another bow, clearly enjoying the adulation.

It was a few minutes before the crowd dispersed and moved away.

Kate realised that Calvin was frowning at her. 'Are you okay?'

'I'm fine.' Embarrassed, she wiped a tear away. 'The cold is making my eyes water.'

She was hardly going to spill the beans about her dad, not when she'd promised herself she wouldn't dump any more emotional baggage on him. The poor man had enough to deal with and didn't need her grief adding to it.

He didn't look convinced, but obviously decided to let it go. 'Shall we look around the grounds? Unless you'd prefer to go back to the house, if you're cold?'

'No, I'm fine. I'd love to look around. It's so pretty.' They moved away from the building and headed through a rose arch covered in cascading white lights. 'Is the story about Ursula true, do you think?'

He gave a half shrug. 'Records confirm the existence of a woman called Ursula Harcourt living at Rose Court during the sixteenth century, and Greystones was a monastery during that time, so it's possible, I guess, but as to whether they were lovers, who knows.'

'I don't like the idea of Ursula not finding peace.'

Calvin stopped walking. 'Kate, you do know the whole ghost thing is nonsense, don't you? Rose Court isn't haunted, it's just in need of repair. The banging windows, the moving objects… It all has a valid explanation.'

'I know that.' She turned away, feeling slightly foolish. 'Doesn't mean I can't allow my imagination to run wild for a moment. Besides, it would make a good film. I'm surprised no one's made one about the place, it could give *A Christmas Carol* a run for its money.' She stopped to admire the apple orchard, pulsating with green lights.

Calvin joined her. 'Talking of films, I watched *It's a Wonderful Life* last night.'

She turned to him. 'You did? Did you enjoy it?'

'It was okay. Not as good as *Home Alone*.'

Her hands went to her hips. 'Calvin Johnson, did you really just say that?'

'What have I said? It's a good film,' he said, defensively.

'It's a *kids'* film.'

'Nothing wrong with that.' He looked put out. 'What's your favourite Christmas film?'

She considered it. '*The Holiday*. Jude Law and Kate Winslet.'

'And you laughed at my film choice?'

'What's wrong with *The Holiday*?' It was her turn to sound defensive.

'It's a *girls'* film.'

She couldn't help laughing. 'Fair enough. Point taken.'

He was grinning. 'Bloody cheek.'

They headed towards the lake and over a small wooden bridge. Strings of fairy lights were wrapped around the posts, forming a canopy of twinkling lights. It struck her that, as well as being Christmassy, it was also very romantic.

They stopped and looked over the edge, watching the water disappearing under the bridge.

Calvin rested his arms on the balustrade. 'What's your favourite Christmas song?'

'Well, I have two... Ella Fitzgerald's version of "The Man with the Bag", which I used to love playing on the piano, and more recently, "Christmas in the Air", by Scouting for Girls. You probably don't know it.'

'Actually, I do.' He straightened up. 'You don't have completely bad taste then. Just in films.'

'From the grown man who still watches *Home Alone*.'

He followed her off the bridge, laughing. 'Woodland or lake?'

She pointed ahead. 'I saw signposts for a magical trail. I like the sound of that.'

They headed towards the woodland, the crowds dispersing as the ground became wetter and heavier. The trees were full of lights and she wondered how on earth anyone could afford the electricity bill for such an elaborate display.

'Wow, look at the reindeer.' The woodland was filled with a herd of glistening wire sculptures, grouped together to form huddles. 'It's so beautiful,' she said, unearthing her phone so she could send some photos to Beth.

They continued walking and reached the start of the magical trail, where only a few brave souls were stoic enough to attempt the route.

As they got closer, Kate could see why. A wooden-slatted walkway had been erected above the forest floor, with rope attached to posts, each one lit by a flickering lantern. It didn't look particularly stable – something that was confirmed when she stepped onto it and it moved beneath her.

Calvin reached for her. 'Careful, it's slippery. Do you want me to go in front so you can hold on to me?'

'Yes, please. Although I can't promise not to bring you down with me.'

He grinned. 'Same here.'

'That's okay, then.' She let him go past and clutched the back of his jacket.

They moved slowly down the walkway, admiring the reindeer and the occasional star dangling from a tree, which shimmered when a blast of light swept across the forest floor.

'You okay back there?'

'Positively peachy,' she said, slipping and smacking into his back. 'Oops, sorry.'

His hand reached around to steady her. 'So, continuing with our festive theme… what's your favourite Christmas food? And please don't say Brussels sprouts.'

'I wasn't going to.' She was briefly distracted when the light show switched to purple, giving the woodland a mythical glow. 'Chinese.'

He glanced over his shoulder. 'That's not a Christmas food.'

'I know, but the first Christmas after Tristan left, my mum was away visiting Brian's family, and I couldn't be bothered to cook,' she said, urging him to continue walking. 'So I ordered in a Chinese, and it sort of became a tradition. Doesn't matter where I end up spending Christmas Day, at some point over the holidays I order myself a takeaway. I guess it's my way of sticking two fingers up to convention.'

He laughed. 'You're such a rebel, Katiekins.'

Was it wrong that she liked him calling her Katiekins? 'What about you? I'm guessing you're a fan of the traditional turkey dinner?'

'Guess again.'

'Roast beef?' Annoyingly, her scarf had become loose and she could feel cold air tickling her neck. 'Goose? Duck?'

He shook his head. 'Indian.'

'Indian?' She stopped walking. 'Having just taken the piss out of me for liking Chinese food at Christmas, you're now telling me you like Indian?'

He turned so he was facing her, his expression amused as he watched her slipping about. 'Seems we have more in common than we thought.'

'I'm not convinced. I need to test this theory further.' She grabbed hold of a post to steady herself. 'Biggest fear?'

He edged closer, careful with his footing. 'You mean, aside from dropping down dead of heart failure?'

'Oh, shit!' Her face fell.

'I'm joking.' He took her scarf from her. 'Besides, you know my biggest fear. Anything creepy-crawly.' He wrapped her scarf around her neck, his fingers brushing against her skin and adding to the goosebumps already present. 'What's your biggest fear?'

'Rings.'

He paused. 'Rings?'

'Weird, I know. But I have this irrational fear that it's going to get stuck on my finger, and I'm not going to be able to get it off, and then my finger starts swelling up and turning blue, and I end up in A & E, where they can't get it off either, and the only solution is to have my finger amputated because it's turned gangrenous and if they don't lop it off, I'll die of sepsis.'

He was fighting a smile. 'That escalated quickly.'

'You asked.'

He tucked her scarf inside her coat, making it snug. 'Didn't you wear a wedding ring when you were married?'

'I tried, but it was a constant cause of argument. He'd get offended if I didn't wear it, and I'd get panicky if I did. Is it any wonder the marriage didn't work?'

'The marriage didn't work because he was a dickhead.' Calvin rested his hands on her shoulders. 'Sorry, but he was.'

'No argument from me.'

His expression softened. 'I find it incredible that he treated someone as lovely and sweet as you are so cruelly. The man is an idiot.' His expression was filled with such compassion that she had to fight the urge to rest her head against his chest. He had such a nice chest. She knew, she'd seen it naked.

'Such is life,' she said with a shrug. 'But I'm done thinking about him. He doesn't deserve my attention.'

'Good decision.'

'We need a less depressing topic. How about this? What's your favourite thing to do? The thing that gives you most pleasure in life?' And then her brain caught up with her mouth. 'Clean answers only,' she said, the cold air failing to disguise the growing heat in her cheeks.

'What are you, a mind reader?' His grin did nothing to ease her embarrassment. 'My favourite thing,' he said, seeming to think it over as his gaze drifted through the trees. 'I'd have to say, that feeling when you get into a steaming hot shower after a freezing game of football. When you're covered in mud and your legs are numb from the cold and you can't feel your hands. I love that burning sensation when the hot water hits your skin and it's so intense, it's almost painful.' He smiled. 'You?'

'Er... toss-up between a foot rub or a head massage.' She wondered if she was revealing too much, but he knew much worse things about her. 'I like having my hair played with.'

Much to her surprise, he gently removed her Christmas-tree hat and slowly ran his hand over her hair in such an intimate way that it felt like he was touching more than just her scalp. 'Like that?' When her eyes drifted shut, he slid his fingers into the hair at the base of her neck and massaged his way up the back of her skull, sending shock waves racing through her.

'Just like that,' she managed, although how, she had no idea.

It was like he'd ignited every nerve ending she possessed. Dormant senses sprang to life, confused and sleepy, as if woken from a long slumber. They raced around her body, disorientated and confused, bumping into each other and staggering about like drunken little elves, wondering what the hell was going on. She could almost imagine her libido yelling through a megaphone, '*This is not a drill! This is not a drill!*'

Frankly, if she hadn't been leaning against the wooden post, she'd have fallen in the water by now. Her legs had lost any strength and her bones had turned to liquid. It had been a long, long time since she'd experienced such tenderness and affection. And it said a lot about the state of her damaged self-esteem that the mere sensation of a man touching her hair could reduce her to a quivering mess. She wasn't sure whether she was embarrassed, turned on or just so bloody grateful she could weep with relief. All three, probably.

His face lowered to hers and he whispered, 'Want me to stop?'

'Hell, no…' Her legs had begun shaking. Helpful. Like she wasn't enough of a mess. 'Although, I should probably admit that I'm so cold I can't actually feel my lips.'

His mouth pressed against hers and it was like a rush of heat so intense and unexpected that she wondered if this was what it was like to be tasered. Maybe not tasered… Whatever the pleasurable equivalent of being tasered might be. She was rambling. Understandably. Calvin Johnson was kissing her. *Kissing her!* His lips were touching hers, his tongue teasing her mouth, his free hand still entangled in her hair and adding to the building heat.

This was the stuff of dreams. Really hot, erotic dreams that she'd never actually managed to turn into reality, but sure as hell wanted to. If her dormant senses were confused before, they were positively humming now.

He gently pulled away, resting his forehead against hers. 'Better?'

She managed a weak nod. 'I get what you mean about the shower thing now.'

Boy, did she.

Chapter Sixteen

Monday, 20th December

Calvin parked up outside the care home and switched off the engine. He didn't immediately get out – he wasn't entirely sure why. Instead, he sat there, gazing at the place he'd reluctantly come to call home, watching the car windows mist over as his breath hit the glass.

It was a gloomy day. The morose building was shrouded in a murky grey mist, mirroring the fog that had settled in his chest and created a dull ache that refused to shift. He should be feeling elated, or at least relieved. Everything he'd hoped to achieve had fallen into place. The probate application had been submitted, he had a buyer lined up for Rose Court and his return to Leeds was imminent. So why did he feel so crap?

Reluctantly, he climbed out of his car and made his way inside.

There was another emotion lurking beneath the surface – one he was reluctant to address – that was adding to his confusion. A feeling that had been niggling at him for a few weeks now, and something that had finally surfaced last night when he'd kissed Kate. It had seemed harmless at the time, effortless and spontaneous, a natural conclusion to a fun evening spent in her company. But in the cold light of day, he knew he had to face the consequences of crossing a line.

He hadn't rationalised his actions at the time; he'd simply allowed himself to fall into the moment and lose himself. The urge to kiss her had snuck up on him, seemingly out of nowhere, and he hadn't resisted temptation. Rational thinking had vanished, replaced by that giddy feeling of physically wanting someone. What followed had taken them both by surprise. Whether it had been the way his body had involuntarily jolted at the unexpectedness of how good it was. Or the way she'd responded with such enthusiasm that they'd both nearly ended up face down in the mud. Or simply that it had reminded him of what he'd been missing and longing for these past few months. Whatever the reason, the end result had been a bittersweet moment that had left him simultaneously craving more and wanting to run a mile.

Either way, he was dreading facing Kate this morning. He'd used the romance and ambience of last night's event to satisfy his own needs, and that wasn't fair. She was vulnerable and grieving, and trying to turn her life around. What she didn't need was him jeopardising her recovery by abusing their friendship and overstepping the mark.

He couldn't imagine she was feeling any better about the situation than he was. He'd put money on her being embarrassed, remorseful or worse – filled with unrealistic expectations about what the future might hold for them. He wasn't up to dealing with any of those scenarios.

He tentatively knocked on the library door, almost hoping to find it empty and her gone. That would certainly let him off the hook. But the idea of never seeing her again caused a wave of panic to flood through him so acutely, that when she called out, 'Come in!' pure relief washed over him.

She was sitting at the desk, wearing her snowmen slippers and typing away on her laptop. The room was warm, thanks to the blazing fire, and there was an unusual sense of calm about the place. He was so used to seeing her flustered, grappling with the stepladders or arguing with the portraits, that it was quite a shock to see her looking relaxed. Her hair was loosely braided and she was wearing a dark-green silky top he hadn't seen before.

She glanced up and smiled. 'Hi, Cal.'

So much for worrying about her emotional state; she seemed fine. He was the one in danger of making a fool of himself.

Other than a faint tint to her cheeks – no doubt due to the heat from the fire rather than any awkwardness – she didn't look out of sorts. In fact, she looked completely composed, like it was just another regular day in the office. She wasn't avoiding eye contact or seemingly embarrassed by his presence. And unlike him, she didn't appear to be resisting the urge to rush over and throw her arms around him.

Any fears he might have had that he'd inadvertently ruined things between them appeared to be unfounded. And he wasn't quite sure how he felt about that.

'I wanted to check you were okay?' he said, using the excuse of removing his jacket to avoid looking directly at her.

'I'm fine,' she said, sounding completely normal. 'Everything okay with you?'

Throwing his jacket on the window seat, he dug his hands in his hoodie pockets. 'Honestly? I'm not sure.'

She swivelled on the office chair to face him. 'Anything I can help with?'

'Maybe.' He gave a brief shrug, chickening out of raising the topic of their kiss and opting for delaying tactics instead. 'I've had a formal offer to buy the care home. I met with the company and their lawyers this morning, and they've given me the contracts to read through.'

Her eyes grew wide. 'It's really happening then?' He couldn't be certain, but he detected a note of disappointment in her voice. 'That was fast, they must be keen.'

'I guess so.' He retrieved the papers from his jacket and walked over to her. 'Would you take a look at the contracts for me and give me your legal opinion?'

'Oh… okay.' Her eyes drifted up to meet his. 'It's not my area of law, but I'll take a look. I'd recommend you engage a solicitor who specialises in commercial law if you decide to go through with the sale, though.'

'Fair enough.' He handed her the contracts, noticing she was wearing little stud earrings that caught in the firelight.

She placed the papers on the desk. 'You know, for someone who's looking at a solution to all their problems, you don't seem very happy.'

'I know. And I don't really understand why.'

'Maybe your gut is trying to tell you something.'

'Maybe.' The dark green of her top suited her skin tone. It was a sheer fabric, with a camisole underneath, and he realised it was the first time she'd worn something that wasn't made of wool and layered her in thick fabrics that disguised her shape.

Was she feeling more comfortable in her skin and no longer felt the need to hide away? Or was it simply that she'd become acclimatised to the lack of decent central heating? Either way, the sight of her pale skin around her neckline wasn't helping to dampen his attraction towards her. The faint outline of her collarbones and the curve of her neck disappearing into her hairline held his gaze. A few loose tendrils of hair had escaped the braid and were curled onto her shoulders, softening the contours of her face.

If anything, he wanted her even more than he had last night, and that was saying something. But it didn't matter how he felt. This wasn't about him – well, not entirely. Whatever his feelings, allowing his emotions to run amok would only hurt her and confuse him – and he was struggling enough as it was. He needed to do the right thing, which meant reining it in.

'I suppose we should talk about what happened last night,' he said, the words tumbling from his mouth before he could censor them.

She sat back and gave him a tentative look. 'I was wondering if you'd bring that up.' The colour in her cheeks intensified, and he knew it had nothing to do with the heat from the fire. 'Part of me thought you might pretend it never happened, and we could avoid the torment of discussing it.'

'I was tempted,' he admitted, feeling his own cheeks growing warm.

'Me too.' A rueful expression appeared on her face.

'The truth is… I enjoyed it… Really enjoyed it. I like spending time with you, and in the heat of the moment, it felt like the right thing to do.'

She let out a long sigh. 'Oh, God, why do I feel like there's a great big but coming.' She rubbed her cheeks. 'I'm not sure my self-esteem can cope with the whole "what seemed like a good idea last night feels wrong this morning" speech, so can we skip the part where you try to let me down gently and just move past it? I'm fine, okay? No permanent damage. I'll survive.'

He was so shocked by her response that it threw him for a moment. He wasn't sure what he'd been expecting, but it wasn't that. 'It didn't feel wrong last night, and I don't regret it this morning—'

'But—' She stood up, her raised hands forming a barrier between them. 'It was still a one-off, right? That's what you're trying to tell me. You have no desire for a repeat performance.' She turned away. 'It's okay, I get it. I'm not dumb enough to think it meant anything.'

Panic raced through him. 'Why would you think it didn't mean anything?'

'Oh, please. Credit me with some intelligence.' She glanced at him, one eyebrow raised. 'Are you telling me it wasn't just a one-off?'

'Well, no, it was… but not because I don't like you…' Or didn't want to do it again, because boy, he did. It had been unbelievably hot, and he wanted nothing more than to pick up where they'd left off. 'But I don't think it would be in either of our best interests to pursue something when we both know it can't go anywhere.'

She closed her eyes. 'You're right… It would be foolish and crazy to start something, especially when I'm leaving in two days' time.'

Her words sent further shock waves racing through him. 'Two days? That soon? But I thought you were staying until after Christmas?'

Her eyes flickered open. 'I would've done if I hadn't managed to get the probate application completed. But there's no need for me to stay now that everything's done, or can be dealt with remotely. No point hanging around.'

He rubbed the back of his neck. 'Right.'

'It's not like there's any reason for me to stay.' Her expression held the glimmer of a challenge, as if she was waiting for him to contradict her.

'I guess not.' He wanted so badly to touch her, especially as he thought he saw a flicker of disappointment skim across her face, but he knew it would only complicate matters. 'And I'll be heading home to Leeds in the new year, assuming the sale goes through, so it's not as if we're going to…' He trailed off, not wanting to admit the truth.

'Have any reason to see each other again?'

He nodded. 'God, that's depressing.'

'No point ignoring reality,' she said, leaning heavily on the chair, as if needing the support. 'Like you said, it's in both our best interests. Besides, neither of us is exactly in the right headspace to offer anything more meaningful at the moment, are we?'

She was right, but far from easing the ache in his chest, the pain only intensified. 'Can we still be friends?'

'Sure.' She nodded, but there was a definite tremor in her hands. 'Friends it is.' She stepped away and forced a smile, her voice conveying more conviction than her body language. 'Now that's sorted, back to business. Do you want the good news or the bad?'

There was so much more he wanted to say, but none of it would have been helpful, so he took her lead and reluctantly accepted the change in topic. 'Good news, please.'

'The garage blocks have sold at auction, so you have another chunk of money available to tide you over until the care-home sale goes through. I transferred the funds this morning.'

She was certainly efficient, he'd give her that.

'Thanks for doing that. I'm planning to offer Nelson a few more shifts, so that'll definitely help. And if I don't book a chiropodist soon, Hanna's threatening to order garden shears and do the job herself. And no one wants that.' He hoped to see her crack a smile, but her expression remained stoically neutral. 'And the bad news?'

'Geraldine got a call from the hospital about her hip replacement operation. They've had a last-minute cancellation, so she's gone off for an assessment appointment with the consultant today.'

He frowned. 'Isn't that good news? I thought she'd be glad to move up the waiting list?'

'In her absence, she's left you with a list of chores to do ahead of the village lantern parade this evening.' She handed him Geraldine's note. 'How are your culinary skills?'

He glanced at the list. 'I have no idea how to make mince pies or mulled wine.'

Kate rubbed her forehead. 'Fine, I'll help you.'

'Are you sure?'

'It's not like I'm busy,' she said, pushing the chair under the desk. 'Like I said, the probate application is done. I'm just tidying up a few things before I leave on Wednesday.'

Wednesday? That was too soon. Far too soon. 'Are you sure you want to help me? After, you know, what we've just discussed?'

She gave him an admonishing look. 'You're not that hot, Calvin Johnson,' she said, placing her hands on her hips. 'Credit me with some restraint.'

He didn't want to tell her it wasn't her restraint he was worried about.

'Besides, can you imagine the grief you'd get from Geraldine if you messed up her kitchen?' She headed over to the door. 'Come on, let's get this over with.'

He followed her into the lobby, wondering why the sinking feeling in his gut hadn't shifted. She'd taken the news better than expected. He'd been worried about upsetting her, but she was fine. In fact, she'd agreed with him. She didn't think starting something was a good idea either. She'd let him off the hook.

So why wasn't he feeling more relieved?

Chapter Seventeen

Tuesday, 21ˢᵗ December

It was the musical notes stencilled on to the door that caught Kate's attention as she scurried along the pavement, shivering from the cold, otherwise she might not have spotted the quaint independent music shop nestled into Ashford's busy High Street. Despite the grandeur of the Georgian building, with its decorative archway, the *Browsers Welcome* sign encouraged her closer. Her train wasn't due for another forty minutes, so she had time for a quick browse.

Hoisting up her Christmas shopping bags, she pushed open the shiny black door, making the bell above jangle. Thankfully, she'd had just enough credit left on her bank card to buy gifts – although she'd stuck to her budget, she was looking forward to a time when she wouldn't have to count every penny. By this time next month, her commission should have come through, and she'd be able to put the past behind her and begin a new phase of her life.

Maybe one day she'd even be able to treat herself to a new piano or guitar. But that was some way off. She needed to find a job first, and that was proving elusive.

As she wandered through the quiet shop, admiring the instruments, she noticed a small soundproof booth. An acoustic guitar was sitting on its stand, its mahogany colouring a reminder of her dad's old Fender Classic.

Checking no one was watching, she slipped inside and shut the door.

Dumping her bags on the floor, she picked up the instrument and trailed her fingers over the strings. It had a nice full sound and her heart pinched at the memory of what she'd lost. There were a lot of things she'd never forgive Tristan for, and selling her dad's guitar definitely secured top spot.

Perching on the stool, she strummed a few chords. She missed playing. Even more, she missed having something that reminded her of her dad. Playing made her feel close to him. Music had been their connection, the trait she'd inherited that kept him alive in her heart.

It had been a while since she'd played, and her fingers felt stiff and clumsy, their tips having softened from a lack of practice. But the muscle memory was still there, and gradually the sound quality improved as she reacquainted herself with the instrument.

It took a few moments for her to recognise the tune her brain had randomly selected: 'Christmas in the Air', by Scouting for Girls. Funny how she'd settled on that particular favourite. Or maybe not so random.

Her mind drifted back to Sunday night and her conversation with Calvin about what they both liked about Christmas. The evening had started out so nicely – it had ended even better. There hadn't been many notable incidents in her life, but kissing Calvin Johnson was a definite highlight. If only she could erase everything that had happened since.

Humming along to the chorus, allowing the music to block out the aftermath of them kissing, she was transported back to that moment. Him stroking her hair, smiling down at her and pulling her into an embrace. She'd been kissed before, of course she had, but she'd never felt consumed the way she had on Sunday evening. It was proper bone-melting stuff. The kind of kiss that swept away inhibitions and ignited a flame that threatened to override any sense of propriety. If that family hadn't appeared on the walkway, she couldn't honestly say what would have happened next.

As it was, the moment had been broken and they'd merged into the crowd, exchanging heated glances as they'd made their way back to Rose Court. The memory had stayed with her all night, preventing sleep, and filling her mind with erotic dreams and images of them rolling about her bed – giving Ursula a run for her money when it came to nightly excursions.

It was only as dawn broke on Monday morning that doubt had started to creep in. Had she overimagined things, and believed it to mean more than it did? As time had ticked away, and with no sign of Calvin, her doubts had morphed into dread. When he'd finally appeared late morning and found her in the library, she'd known what was coming even before he'd uttered a single word. It was the look on his face. She knew regret when she saw it.

Her phone vibrated in her coat pocket and she stopped playing. She had a WhatsApp message from Beth, accompanied by two photos.

Instagram Megan vs Reality Megan.

In the first photo, Megan looked gorgeous in a fitted black dress, showing off her baby bump. Her red lips were pouting at the camera, and her smoky dark eyes were sultry and smouldering. The second photo was a shot of her kneeling on the bathroom floor, with her head over the toilet.

Poor Megan. But feeling sorry for her cousin didn't stop the tears surfacing, and for a moment Kate held her breath, tying to stem the onset. Crying was one thing, giving into a full-blown panic attack was another.

Wiping her eyes, she placed the guitar on its stand, the desire to play eradicated by a wave of sadness. She wasn't sure whether it was missing her dad, thinking about Calvin or the images of Megan's pregnancy that had unsettled her. Either way, she'd lost her battle to remain composed.

Collecting her things, she scurried from the music shop. So much for a nice festive day of shopping and not dwelling. She'd failed spectacularly.

She stepped onto the street and it took her a moment to realise that the wet on her face wasn't just from tears, but from falling snow.

Glancing up, she was met with a darkening sky and a flurry of flakes floating through the air. She'd only been inside the shop a short while, but daylight had faded into dusk.

Shivering, she pulled up the hood on her coat and headed for the train station, her feet aching from a long day wandering around the shops. It hadn't taken long to complete her shopping, but she'd been in no hurry to return to Rose Court.

If facing Calvin yesterday hadn't been excruciating enough, she'd been forced to spend the rest of the afternoon with him, baking mince pies and brewing a huge vat of mulled wine for last night's village lantern parade. Even though deep inside she'd known the kiss was a one-off, a moment of madness that hadn't meant anything, a small part of her had clung on to the idea that just maybe it was the start of something magical between them. But it was just another disappointment in a long line of disappointments. He'd been extraordinarily kind and let her down gently, but the rejection still stung.

Of course, she hadn't let him see that. She had some pride, and there was no way she was going to embarrass herself further by admitting she was hoping for a repeat performance. Instead, she'd reverted to business mode, put Christmas music on the kitchen radio and busied herself cooking, so she wouldn't have to keep looking at his tantalisingly inviting lips and wishing they were still attached to hers.

It was a sound plan, almost flawless, and it did a pretty decent job of keeping her emotions in check… until he'd encountered a large spider in the larder and reacted as though the entire inhabitants of Jurassic Park had escaped their pens and were chasing him around the kitchen.

In their efforts to trap the spider, a bag of flour had been upturned, covering them both in white dust, and resulting in uncontrollable laughter and flawed attempts to clean each other up.

It was at this point she'd decided her resolve had been stretched to breaking point, and if she didn't escape soon, she'd be in danger of grabbing him, pushing him onto the kitchen table and straddling him. Something that, although highly appealing, would only exacerbate the awkwardness between them. So she did the sensible thing and ran to her room, where she'd been hiding ever since, counting down the hours until she could escape back to her family in Surrey.

Not that she had anything to go back to. With a groan, she recalled Beth's phone call and stumbled to a halt. Hearing the news that her Christmas plans had been scuppered had only added to her gloom. She was not destined to have a 'Happy Christmas' this year.

Checking the road for cars, she was about to cross when she saw a sign for Ashford's Legal Clinic. The sign directed her towards the station, so she followed it, figuring she had a few minutes to spare before her train was due.

The clinic was a generic office space squashed between a bakery and a hardware shop.

Intrigued, she pushed open the door and was greeted by a woman sitting behind a desk.

The woman removed her glasses. 'Good afternoon. Do you have an appointment to see one of our solicitors?'

Kate pushed the hood of her coat down. 'I was just passing and saw the sign. I didn't realise there was a legal clinic in Ashford.'

'We haven't been here that long. The place was set up by local family law solicitor Yvette Bond,' the woman said, handing Kate a business card. 'Four solicitors are now regularly using the facilities.'

Kate glanced around. 'Using the facilities? In what way?'

'We run a rent-a-chair scheme. You know, like the hair salons do. Although in our case, it's rent an office. The solicitors work from home on a self-employed basis, but they book an office when they need to see a client. It keeps the costs down and saves them having to rent permanent office space.'

Kate placed her bags on the floor. 'I've never heard of solicitors renting an office before.'

'Are you in the legal profession?'

'I'm a wills and probate solicitor.' Even though she didn't feel particularly professional, standing there in her thick coat, woollen scarf and fluffy Ugg boots.

'Then you might be interested in our Wishing Will scheme.' The woman reached across for a flyer. 'Yvette has been struggling to find a local solicitor willing to cover the Ashford area. It's a scheme to enable people without means to draft a will.'

Kate took the flyer. 'Pro bono, you mean?'

'Not exactly. The solicitor drafts the will free of charge, but the fee is included in the document, so it forms part of the estate when the person dies. Of course, most of our clients don't have large estates, so invariably the bill never gets paid, which is why it doesn't appeal to most solicitors. No money to be made. Or not much, anyway.'

'I can see that. But it sounds like a great scheme.' Kate could think of several people who had enquired about making a will when she'd worked for Blandy & Kite but who couldn't afford the fees upfront.

The woman tilted her head. 'I don't suppose you'd be interested in taking part?'

Kate smiled. 'I'd love to, but I'm only in the area temporarily.'

'That's a shame. Who do you work for?'

'No one at the moment. I've just finished dealing with a local estate, and now I'm on the hunt for a full-time job.'

'How's it going?'

'Not great so far,' she admitted, her confidence dented with each rejection. 'I've applied for a few positions, but no interviews as yet. It's early days, so I'm sure something will come up.'

The woman gave her an appraising look. 'Have you considered working for yourself?'

'Self-employed, you mean?'

'It works for the solicitors we have using the space here. They like the freedom to manage their own hours and workloads, without the pressure to hit targets.'

'That's the bit I hate,' Kate said, searching her pockets for a tissue. 'Billing a grieving widow for time spent with them talking about their dead husband never sat comfortably.'

'Maybe you should consider it, then.' The woman offered her a box of tissues. 'Be your own boss.'

'Oh, thanks.' Kate took a tissue, noticing the time when she glanced at the wall clock. 'Oh, heavens, my train! I need to go. Thanks for the information. It's been really interesting.'

'My pleasure. And good luck with the job hunting!' the woman called after her, as Kate almost fell out the door.

Waving a goodbye, Kate ran towards the station, praying she wouldn't miss her train. It was too cold to be standing on a platform waiting for the next one, especially as the snow was coming down harder now.

Lifting her bags over the barrier, she just made it onto the platform as the train pulled into the station. It was rush hour so it was full and there were no spare seats. Edging her way through the packed carriage, she ended up standing by the doors, her shoulder pressed against the glass.

Thankfully, it was only a short ride to Pluckley. She rested her head against the door, her mind processing the information the woman had given her. Should she consider going it alone as a solicitor? She loved her work, but she hated targets. Was this really something she could do?

The idea of being her own boss certainly appealed. Working at Rose Court had been a breath of fresh air – well, if you discounted the cold conditions, wayward ghosts, eccentric residents and falling for the man who had hired her. Aside from that, it had been perfect.

But she had nowhere to live. No savings. No way of setting herself up. Realistically, she'd need capital to get herself started, and she didn't have that.

Her heart sank. It was a lovely idea, but probably not possible at this moment in time. Maybe one day, when she was more settled and financially stable. Until then, she was better off finding regular employment.

The train braked so suddenly, she almost lost her balance.

Grabbing the handrail, she peered outside and spotted the faded sign for Pluckley, disappearing under a blanket of snow.

When she stepped off the train, she was hit by a gust of icy air blowing down the platform. The temptation to phone Calvin and ask for a lift was overwhelming. Especially when she remembered his heated seats and cosy blanket stored in the boot. But seeing him wouldn't help and being in a car with him would only make matters worse. She was better off fighting the cold and suffering physically rather than emotionally.

As she headed away from the station and into the snowy dark night, a sense of déjà vu settled over her, as she remembered her first night in Pluckley. So much had happened since then. Most of it good. She'd successfully completed the probate submission, her panic attacks had reduced, and her plan to pay off the tax debt and avoid bankruptcy looked to be on track. She should be feeling elated. If only she wasn't facing Christmas alone, she had a job to ensure her recovery continued and she hadn't stupidly fallen for Calvin bloody Johnson. But that's what happened when you let your guard down.

A set of headlights approaching forced her to step onto the grassy verge to avoid being mowed down. The soft wet ground squelched beneath her feet, soaking her furry boots.

The car braked hard and reversed to where she was standing.

Even before the window lowered, she knew it would be Calvin, as she'd recognised his flashy car. Her luck had run out in trying to avoid him.

He leant across and opened the door. 'Get in,' he said, not unkindly.

'I'm okay walking,' she replied, a feeble attempt to retain her dignity.

His expression conveyed what he thought about her refusal. 'Don't be daft. It's freezing out there. Please get in.' His voice softened, and she knew only a fool would refuse for the sake of wounded pride.

Resigned to her situation, she climbed in, passing over her shopping bags so he could place them on the back seat. The heating was on, and her senses went into overdrive as she breathed in his familiar musky scent. Of course he smelt good, why was she even surprised.

'Just as well I saw you,' he said, pulling away. 'Why didn't you call me for a lift?'

'I didn't want to bother you, and the weather wasn't this bad when I left Ashford.'

He turned the heated seats up a notch, no doubt noticing her shivering. 'How was your shopping trip? Did you get everything you needed?'

'I did, thanks.' She briefly considered telling him about the music shop and the legal clinic, but decided against sharing any further personal information with him. She'd divulged too much as it was. That was how she'd got into this mess in the first place. She'd opened up and let him in, and look where it had got her – feeling like a prized numpty. She needed to steer the conversation towards safer ground. 'Are you heading out somewhere? I assume you weren't randomly driving about looking for me?'

'I'm meeting up with Nelson in Ashford,' he said, adjusting his baseball cap – now minus the reindeer. 'I kept a lookout in case I saw you. I figured you'd be returning soon.' His concern for her did nothing to ease her attraction towards him. Why couldn't he be a selfish arse? It would make life so much easier.

'Boys' night out, huh?'

'Something like that.' A pause followed, as if he was tentative about admitting something. 'He's invited me to training night at his football club.'

She knew this was a big deal, but she also knew he wouldn't appreciate a fuss. 'Are you going to join in?'

He shook his head. 'Just watch.'

She searched for something encouraging to say. 'It'll be nice for you to hang out with a few blokes your own age for once.'

He laughed. 'Esme said the same thing.'

God, she'd missed his laugh.

'Shame you'll miss the Christmas singalong,' she said, trying to cover the turmoil bubbling inside her. 'I thought you'd enjoy belting out a few Bing Crosby numbers.'

'Maybe another time,' he said, smiling. Thankfully, it was dark and she couldn't see the full impact of his dimples. 'At least I'll escape Geraldine trying to dance with me.' He glanced over. 'What about you? Will you join them?'

'For a while, but I have to pack. I'm off first thing.'

The car seemed to slow for no apparent reason. 'You're definitely leaving then?' His voice was barely a whisper.

'That's the plan.' It was pretty impressive how together she sounded. Like her leaving was no big deal and wouldn't cause her any physical pain whatsoever.

'I wondered if your plans might've changed,' he said, as they passed through the village. 'I was chatting to Alex earlier and he said he's staying at Rose Court for Christmas, as there's no one at home.'

She silently cursed her cousin for spilling the beans about their change of plans.

'Well, that's true,' she said, searching for a way of avoiding the truth… and failing. 'Beth and her partner Matt are spending the day with his mum and sister. Megan is visiting Zac's family, and Uncle Kenneth is taking his girlfriend Tiffany to the Maldives. Aunty Connie was planning to stay at home but then she heard about the Maldives trip and has now booked herself on a

Caribbean cruise. She doesn't like it when her ex-husband tries to outdo her. Still, I don't blame her, a holiday sounds lovely.'

Calvin was quiet for a moment. 'Weren't you supposed to be spending the holidays with your mum?'

She blew into her chilly hands, wishing she didn't have to reveal what had happened. 'I was, but Brian's mum had a fall yesterday and broke her hip. She's booked in for surgery tomorrow and she'll be in hospital for a few days, so they need to stay up there and look after her.'

Her poor mum had sounded so upset when she'd called earlier. She hated the idea of her daughter being left alone for Christmas, but Kate had assured her it was fine, and they'd get together soon. Such was life.

'Where does that leave you?' he said, pulling into the care-home driveway. 'Who will you spend Christmas with?'

'Not sure yet.' She focused on the gargoyle statues, which were looking particularly ominous tonight. 'Beth and Megan said I can join them for their respective gatherings, so I have options. It's not like I'll be on my own,' she lied, hoping he wouldn't detect the tremble in her voice.

Her cousins had genuinely made the offer, but Kate didn't feel up to socialising with other people's families this year. She wanted her own family. And if she couldn't have that, she'd rather be on her own.

'You could always stay at Rose Court?' he said, slowing the car to a stop.

She unclicked her seat belt. 'Thanks, but I don't think that's a good idea.'

'Why not?' He shifted his body to face her. 'Because I messed up?'

'You didn't mess up,' she assured him, wondering how she'd managed to get the seat belt stuck in her coat zip.

'Of course I did. We were getting on fine, becoming really good friends, and then I blew it.' He rubbed his forehead. 'I'm such an idiot. I'm so sorry, Kate.'

215

'It wasn't all you,' she said, struggling to unhook her blessed seat belt. 'It's not like I was fighting you off. It was my fault as much as yours.'

'But I hate that it's made things awkward between us.' He caught her arm, stopping her from wrestling with the seat belt. 'Please don't leave on my account. Everyone will be really sad to see you go, they adore you.'

She couldn't look at him. 'I think it's better if I leave.'

'I wish you wouldn't,' he said softly, sounding so upset that she nearly caved, and that wouldn't have been sensible. Her fragile heart couldn't take another knock-back.

With a sigh, he unhooked her seat belt and let it slide away. She opened the car door. 'Thanks for the lift.'

'Will I see you in the morning, before you go?'

'Sure,' she said, but she fully intended to be long gone before anyone awoke. She'd say her goodbyes tonight and then scurry away, tail between her legs. 'It's not like I won't be in touch. We'll need to chat in January to arrange the transfer of assets and pay the beneficiaries.'

'Right.' He nodded slowly. 'I'll pay your bill as soon as the money hits my account.'

'I'd appreciate that. I'll email you my invoice, so you know what the final total is.'

Silence descended. 'So, that's it?'

'That's it. Enjoy your football training.' She slid out of the car like a cowardly snake, hating the way every nerve ending in her body was screaming at her to stay.

What would be the point? She'd have to leave some time, and it was better to get it over and done with than prolong the agony.

'Night,' she said, grabbing her shopping bags and running up the care-home steps. Her throat was tight and tears threatened, but she forced herself to keep it together, determined that he wouldn't see her cry.

The music hit her the moment she entered the lobby. The door to the lounge was open and she could see Lucky Larry at the piano. He was playing 'When a Child is Born', his voice low and raspy. Rowan and Esme were arm in arm, swaying, looking glassy-eyed and slightly drunk, and Natalie was cradling Jacob. Even Hanna was there, the only one not wearing a festive outfit, although her blue-black hair did have sprinkles of glitter in it. Alex was watching her, an odd look on his face, as if he was part-transfixed, part-terrified.

Kate was going to miss these people. She hadn't meant to get attached, but they felt like family now.

'Ah, here you are!' Geraldine said, exiting the kitchen and startling her. 'We were wondering where you'd got to. Have you eaten?'

The mention of food made her tummy rumble. 'I'll grab something later,' she said, not wanting to encroach on Geraldine's fun. 'You go and join the others. I can sort myself out.'

'No need,' she said, smiling. 'Calvin left you something in the kitchen. It'll need heating up in the microwave, but it might still be warm enough. Come and join us when you're done. No arguments, okay? You're part of the team now.'

Calvin had left her something? 'Er… I will, I promise.' She headed into the kitchen, intrigued.

A paper bag was sitting on the table, her name scribbled on it. Next to it was a note and a wrapped gift. She read the note.

Just ensuring you get your Christmas Chinese.
Love, Cal. X

Kate peered inside the bag, breathing in a waft of ginger, spices and peanut satay. He'd bought her a Chinese takeaway? What the hell was he trying to do to her?

Ignoring the shake in her hands, she picked up the gift and peeled away the wrapping. Inside was a DVD. *The Holiday.*

Sinking onto a chair, her head dropped onto the table with a loud thud.

So much for holding it together.

Chapter Eighteen

Wednesday, 22nd December

Calvin winced when the loud buzzing of the hair clippers sent shock waves vibrating through his skull. He couldn't remember the last time he'd had a hangover. Thankfully, he'd downed a pint of water before collapsing into bed last night, so the effects of consuming too many bottles of Peroni weren't as crippling as they might have been.

What had started out as a quiet evening, watching football training, had ended up with a group visit to a curry house in Ashford, followed by a few pints at The Black Horse Inn with Nelson. His car was still parked outside the pub, which had seemed sensible at the time, but less so when they were staggering home in the drifting snow. There was no way of retrieving the car this morning, as two feet of snow were blocking the driveway.

On the plus side, the heavy snowfall meant that the local trains weren't running, so Kate hadn't been able to leave as planned and was trapped at Rose Court, along with everyone else. Thank heavens for small mercies. Although he wasn't quite sure she saw it that way.

Lucky Larry appeared from his bathroom, a towel tucked into the collar of his blue shirt. 'Ready when you are.'

'Are you sure you about this?' Calvin had a definite shake in his hands.

Larry sat down at the dressing table. 'I need a haircut and won't be getting into town anytime soon in this weather, so clipper away. What's the worst that can happen?'

Calvin winced. 'I make a mess of it?'

'It looks the same whether it's a good or bad cut. And with my eyesight, I can't tell the difference.' He met Calvin's reflection in the mirror. 'Besides, you're more used to handling Afro hair than anyone else here. You've been selected by default.'

Calvin picked up the wide-tooth comb. 'Don't say I didn't warn you.'

Larry smiled. 'How was soccer training last night? Looks like it involved liquor.'

'It did.' Calvin winced. 'And I'm feeling the effects this morning.'

'Do I need to do a sobriety test? How many heads do I have?'

Calvin squinted into the mirror. 'Just the one... I think.'

Larry laughed. 'Okay, then. You know, I'd get so blasted in my day that I couldn't tell the black keys from the white ones. Probably accounts for why I can still play piano with poor eyesight. I'm used to blurred vision.'

Calvin combed through Larry's hair. He was struggling to cope with one hangover, let alone having to deal with them on a regular basis. He supposed it was part of being a musician. The collection of framed Motown discs hanging on Larry's bedroom wall was a reminder of the man's prestigious career. 'Did you drink a lot when you were younger?'

'Sure, it was all part of the scene back then. The band wouldn't come on stage until nine and we never finished before one in the morning. You'd be too hyped to sleep, so you'd unwind with a few shots at the bar and then sleep it off the next day. That was my life for many years, until I met my Francie. Things change when you have a reason to get up in the morning. You get my drift?'

Calvin picked up the clippers. 'I do.'

'You have that in your life?'

'Not anymore.' Calvin searched through the range of guards, trying not to think about his fractured love-life, past or present. 'Number four okay?'

'Perfect.' He could feel Larry watching him as he fitted the guard to the clippers. 'I kinda thought you might be sweet on Kate. She's quite a gal, you know. I like her.'

'I like her, too,' he admitted, knowing there was no point denying it. He wasn't oblivious to the sly looks when they were together and the muted conversations that would abruptly stop when he entered a room. It seemed everyone at Rose Court had known what was going on long before they had. And now it was over. Ended before it had even started, and all because he'd been an idiot.

'If I was fifty years younger, I might make a play for her myself,' Larry said, with a wink.

Calvin ran the clippers up the back of Larry's head. 'You'd probably be more successful. You have more in common with her than I do – she's very passionate about music.'

'Seems to me she's passionate about a lot of things. I see kindred spirits.'

Calvin raised an eyebrow. 'Hardly.'

'You don't feel a connection?'

'Maybe, but it's… complicated.' He didn't want to say too much, as it wouldn't be fair on Kate. Whatever was going on between them needed to remain private.

Larry tilted his head. 'How so?'

'Bad timing, mainly… keep your head still,' he said, fearful of taking a chunk out of Larry's ear. 'This is precarious enough as it is.'

'What do you mean, bad timing? You either like each other, or you don't. There's nothing complicated about it.'

If only that was true, but life wasn't that simple. He wished it was.

Realising Larry was waiting for an answer, he chose his words carefully. 'We've both recently come out of long-term relationships, and we're trying to rebuild our careers. I don't think either of us is in the right frame of mind to start something new with someone else.'

Larry seemed to ponder this, as Calvin resumed shaving the back of his head. 'You know, when I met my Francie, she'd just got divorced. Bad marriage to a bad man, who'd destroyed her confidence and left her with two broken fingers.'

Calvin frowned. 'Nice man.'

'He was a jerk, that's for sure. When I saw her at the club that first night, waitressing, she was so sad she wouldn't even lift her eyes to mine. I wanted to whisk her off and marry her that very day.'

Calvin stopped shaving. 'And did you?'

He shook his head. 'It took months of persuading. I'd walk her home each night after her shift and tell her I loved her. The following day I'd show up with a single rose and ask her to marry me. I did that every day for six months and every day she'd turn me down. Said she was too damaged and no good for me, I could do better, and she was doing me a favour refusing me.' Larry looked wistful as his eyes drifted to the dressing table and the sepia photo of his wife. 'But I knew she was the gal for me, and I wasn't gonna stop asking until she agreed to marry me. Deep down inside, you see, I knew it was meant to be.'

Calvin resumed cutting. 'How did you know?'

'Gut instinct.' Larry patted his stomach. 'That feeling you get when you know something's worth fighting for.'

'And she eventually said yes?'

'Hell, yes. Happiest day of my life. Hers, too. Years later she told me she'd wanted to say yes from the beginning, but she didn't trust I was being genuine. She didn't feel worthy of love and felt it was too good to be true.'

Calvin angled the clippers around Larry's ear. 'What changed her mind?'

'She had this bad dream one night about lying in an old folks' home on her deathbed, with no loved ones, and she realised she didn't want that. She'd rather risk another heartbreak than spend her days alone.'

Calvin blew on the clippers to disperse the loose hair. 'So it worked out in the end?'

'We were married for over thirty years.' Larry glanced at the photo again, his face easing into a smile. 'What d'you think?'

Calvin smiled, too. 'Persistence won out, huh?'

'It was more about trusting my instincts. Some relationships aren't always perfect, they start out in the wrong place, or at the wrong time. But maybe that's what makes them work, because you have to battle through the hard stuff to get to the happy ending. It makes the reward that much sweeter.'

'You're an old romantic, you know that, Larry?'

'I'm a blues musician, we all are,' he said, with a wry smile. 'You decided whether you're staying at Rose Court yet?'

Calvin moved to Larry's other side. 'Not yet.'

'What's holding you back? Don't you enjoy looking after us old folk?'

'It's not that. I don't mind the work, and I like the staff and residents. I just don't think care work is my calling.'

Larry met his eyes in the mirror. 'How d'you figure that?'

'If it wasn't for Hanna and Natalie, I'd be lost. Without them the place wouldn't survive. I don't have the knowledge or experience to run a care home. It's not fair on the residents to have someone in charge who isn't trained to do the job. I need to find something I'm good at.'

'Like soccer, you mean?'

'Exactly.' Calvin gave one last sweep over Larry's head, checking he hadn't missed anything. 'I knew how to play football, what was expected of me, and I felt confident in my abilities.'

'Of course you did – you'd been doing it long enough, you'd had time to develop and build your skills. All that training and being coached meant that by the time you stepped onto that pitch as a professional player, you were up to the task. You think you'd have been as good if you hadn't had that time to develop and learn your craft?'

'Of course not.' Calvin unclipped the guard. 'Tilt your head forwards so I can tidy up your neck.'

'So why do you expect to be proficient at running a care home when you're brand new to it? I hate to break it to you, son, but whatever career you go into, you'll be starting at the bottom. It'll take time and patience for you to learn a new skill. There's no shortcut, or bypassing hard work and commitment. The sooner you accept that, the easier it'll be.'

Calvin sighed. As depressing as it was, the man had a point. He hated feeling like an amateur; he wanted to feel the heady heights of success he'd felt as a footballer. But expecting to step straight into another job at the same level was naive.

'You want my advice? Pick something that makes you feel good about yourself and gives you a sense of satisfaction. Then work out how to get better at it. Go to college, do an online course, whatever it takes to obtain the skills you need. You've too many years ahead of you to be stuck in a job you hate.'

Calvin brushed away the loose hair from Larry's neck. 'You're a wise man, Larry.'

'I have my moments. Now, let's look at this haircut.' He peered into the mirror, angling his head. 'Looks good, son.'

'Glad you like it.' Calvin unplugged the clippers and placed them back in the box.

'And just for the record, I think you're great at managing this place. You know why? You don't treat us like we're past it. You show us kindness and dignity, and you allow us the freedom to be independent and self-sufficient. As much as we can be, anyway.' Larry pushed himself up from the stool. 'It's not a great feeling getting older and realising you can't do the things you used to do. Hell, some days I can't even remember why I walked into a room. It's scary when you realise you're at the front of the train and the next stop is the morgue.'

Calvin looked at the man's mournful expression.

'Everyone here had another life before this. A life that we still desperately want, but can no longer have, where we were capable and independent, and masters of our own universe. Accepting you no longer have the life you want is a blow like no other. And you, more than anyone, know what that feels like… right, son?'

The lump in Calvin's throat prevented him from speaking.

'You give us hope that, just maybe, the time we have left might not be quite so dull as we feared. Who else would let us get blasted and go on village excursions to the pub?'

Despite smiling, Calvin felt riddled with guilt. He doubted the new owners would allow that to continue. They offered a full range of activities, from seated exercise to painting for beginners, but nowhere did it mention participating in local ghost hunts and organising Fuzzy Duck drinking games.

Larry reached up and patted Calvin's cheek. 'This is your calling, son. I can feel it in my gut, just like I knew it with my Francie. And despite what you say, you don't suck at it as much as you think.' Larry shuffled over to the bed. 'Time for my lie-down. I like to party with the rest of them, but some of us oldies also need our rest.'

Calvin left Larry's room, mulling over the older man's words. He was right. Whatever Calvin did next, he'd be starting from scratch. He'd be a novice, an apprentice, relegated to the bottom rung. It was a depressing thought. But was Larry right when he said that managing Rose Court was his calling? That bit he wasn't so certain about.

Trying to fathom his life with a foggy head probably wasn't the best idea, so he pushed the thought away and decided to check on Kate.

He hadn't seen her all day, and he could only imagine how she felt about being trapped here. He'd still been asleep when she'd attempted to leave this morning, and according to Geraldine, she'd headed off down the driveway with her suitcase dragging behind her, only to return a few minutes later when she'd realised the lanes were completely blocked.

Since then she'd been holed up in her room and no one had seen her. He hated the idea of her being miserable.

Heading up to the second floor, he knocked tentatively on her closed bedroom door, hoping she wouldn't yell at him to go away.

When no one answered, he knocked harder. Still no response.

'Kate? Are you okay? I'm worried about you.'

Still no answer.

Twisting the handle, he gently pushed the door. 'Kate…? Are you in here?'

No sign of her.

The bed was stripped, her bulging suitcase sat on the floor, unpacked, and her possessions were missing from the side table. She hadn't given up on the idea of leaving, then?

The window rattled suddenly and flew open, startling him.

There was no wind today, so why the window had randomly opened, he had no idea. As he went over to close it, he spotted Kate in the neighbouring field, walking up an incline, dragging something large behind her.

When she reached the top, she turned around and straddled what looked like a tray and sat on top of it. Pushing herself away, she only travelled a few feet before toppling into the snow. She was sledging?

Shaking his head in bemusement, he secured the window and left her room. He'd be glad when they had enough money to fix the bloody thing. But whether he'd be the one dealing with the repairs, or whether it would be the new owners, he wasn't sure. He had no idea how long the sale would take. That's if he decided to sell.

Ignoring the confusion of thoughts running through his head, he made his way downstairs and picked up his jacket, before venturing outside.

The depth of the snow made wading through it hard work. It took him a few minutes to reach Kate and in that time she'd attempted another couple of sledge runs, and fallen off both times.

When he finally reached her, he was panting. 'This is not what I expected to find you doing.'

'I needed an outlet for my frustrations,' she said, dragging the tray up the incline. 'And this seemed preferable to having another meltdown. I like to think I've evolved,' she said, positioning the tray between her legs. 'Although, in truth, this isn't as rewarding as I'd hoped it would be.' Her cheeks were glowing from the exertion and her knitted gloves were caked in snow. She looked bulky, unathletic and adorable.

'Hard work?'

'It's exhausting,' she said, sitting heavily on the tray. 'And my bum hurts.' She pushed away and immediately fell off, landing face down in the snow. Laughing, she rolled onto her back. 'Something tells me I might've run out of steam.'

He went over and sat down next to her. 'Sorry you weren't able to escape this morning.'

'I did try.'

'So I heard.' He gave her a nudge. 'You promised me you wouldn't leave without saying goodbye.'

She turned to look at him. 'Rumour has it you got legless last night. I didn't think you'd appreciate an early wake-up call this morning.'

'I wasn't legless… but you're right, I did have a few beers.'

She propped herself onto her elbows. 'Good night?'

He nodded. 'Surprisingly so. They're a nice bunch of lads, and I had fun.' The wet was starting to creep through his jeans. 'Can I have a go?' he said, pointing at the metal tray.

'Go for it.' She manoeuvred herself into a sitting position. 'What was the club like?'

'Big,' he said, dragging himself to his feet. 'As well as the men's teams, they have several kids' teams, two women's teams and a walking football team for the seniors. There was a lot of football going on.' He straddled the tray and sat down.

'Is Nelson any good?'

Calvin recalled the sight of Nelson's exuberant goal celebration after scoring a penalty. 'Better than some of the players on

226

his team.' He pushed away and skidded a few feet, before falling off. 'Well, that was unsatisfactory.'

'Tell me about it.' She rolled her eyes. 'Although I do appreciate you failing at it, too, so I feel less inadequate.'

He grinned. 'I'm kind like that.'

'The ultimate gentleman.' She grinned back. 'Did anyone recognise you at the club?'

He carried the tray up the incline. 'Yeah, despite me trying to keep a low profile. They were mostly cool about it. By the time we'd gone for a beer and a curry, the novelty had worn off and I was just one of the lads.'

'Did you offer them any coaching tips?'

He shook his head. 'Although I did have to stop myself shouting instructions at the kids with disabilities training.' He sat on the tray, determined to make a better go of his second run. 'They don't have a coach and at the moment they're left to run about like headless chickens.'

'I'm sure they'd have appreciated the tips.'

'Maybe.' He pushed away and managed to travel a bit further, before falling off. 'This is harder than it looks.'

'I blame the equipment.' Kate moved her arms and legs about, creating a snow angel. 'A kitchen lap-tray isn't up to the task.'

'I think you might be right. One more attempt and I'm conceding defeat.'

Kate rolled onto her side. 'Has it made you think more about coaching as a career?'

'There's no money to be made from coaching, unless you do it at the highest level,' he said, dragging himself to his feet. 'It would take years to reach the top. But I might consider it as a hobby. Didn't you say I needed to find an interest away from playing?'

She rested her head on her hand. 'Nice to know you listen to me sometimes.'

'I listen to you all the time,' he said, striding up the incline. 'But if I was serious about it, then I'd want to know more about how to coach those kids. I don't know enough about adapting the training to fit different physical abilities.'

Her gaze turned inquisitive. 'Is that something you might be interested in doing?'

'I don't know for certain, but it's the first thing I've felt mildly excited about since I stopped playing.'

'Well, that's got to count for something. And I'm sure you'll find plenty of stuff online about coaching courses.'

'Maybe.' He pushed away and skidded down the incline, gaining some speed, before the tray hit a bump and he was sent flying. 'You know, this isn't the smartest thing to be doing with a hangover.'

'It's much more fun watching you do it. It makes for a great spectator sport.'

He brushed wet snow from his backside. 'So how was your night?'

'Good, thanks.' She shuffled onto all fours in an effort to stand up. 'I ate my Chinese in the lounge, while listening to Esme and Rowan murdering a few Christmas songs, and then headed off to bed to watch *The Holiday*.' She made it to her feet, and began jigging up and down to dislodge the loose snow. 'You didn't have to do that, by the way.'

'I wanted to,' he said, walking over. 'A feeble attempt at an apology.'

'No apology necessary. But thanks, anyway, it was a lovely gesture and I enjoyed the film. I can now tick off Christmas Chinese from my list.' She wiped her mouth, and then grimaced when she realised she'd left bits of wool stuck to her lip-gloss. 'You've had your Christmas Indian, too, so we're all good. All you need now is to watch *Home Alone* and you're sorted.'

He wanted so badly to remove a strand of wool from her lips, but knew the gesture would be too intimate. 'You almost managed to say that without sounding sarcastic.'

She removed her glove and wiped her mouth. 'No judgement here. After all, you did point out that my choice of film was for *girls*.'

He laughed. 'And you said my choice was for *kids*.'

'Well, it is.' She smiled and he was hit by the force of it. When had she become so pretty? Or had he just not been paying attention? 'Are we heading inside now? Only, I'm freezing.'

He forced his gaze away from her lips. 'Fine by me.'

She began walking, her arms outstretched as she tried to remain upright. 'By the way, I've read through the sale contracts.'

He caught her arm when she wobbled. 'What did you think?'

'They look fairly standard as contracts go, nothing too alarming. Except for one thing. The purchase only refers to the physical aspects of the business, like the building and equipment. It doesn't talk about buying the business as a running concern. There's no mention of TUPE.'

He frowned at her. 'What's that when it's at home?'

'Transfer of Undertakings. It's when one company takes over the running of another and the business continues to function with the use of existing staff.'

He stopped walking. 'They're not offering to do that?'

'It doesn't look like it.'

'What does that mean for our staff?'

'Redundancy, unfortunately. It won't be a problem for Geraldine, as she's retiring anyway, but I doubt it'll be good news for Natalie and Hanna. They've put so much effort into keeping everything going.'

She was right. This was not welcome news. 'When I met with the company, they never said they wouldn't be taking on the existing staff team. I just assumed they would.'

'I imagine the new company will need additional staff, so there's no reason why they can't apply for new roles. They're both experienced nurses and I'm sure you'll give them a glowing reference.'

'Of course,' he said, although somehow he doubted that would be enough to ease his guilt. Or their disgruntlement.

He could imagine Hanna's fury. And he didn't even want to think about how upset Natalie would be.

Kate looked uncomfortable. 'Sorry to be the bearer of bad news.'

'It's not your fault. I'm glad you told me.' He was hit by a simultaneous wave of sadness and annoyance. He couldn't help feeling like the company had deliberately misled him.

'Tough decision, huh?'

'Even tougher now. I was already having doubts, and this has made things ten times worse.'

It wasn't just the staff he was worried about. Larry's words – about how great it was that Calvin didn't treat them as if they were incapable of making their own decisions – came back to haunt him. He'd hoped the new company would honour that ethos, but now he wasn't so sure. And that didn't sit comfortably.

Kate tugged on his sleeve. 'Are you okay?'

'Not really. I have no idea what to do. It all feels so over-whelming.' The weight in his chest gripped, intensifying the sense of responsibility he felt.

It was a while before she spoke. 'You know… maybe you should talk to someone about it.'

He frowned. 'I am talking to someone – I'm talking to you.' She was the only person he could open up to. He didn't even want to think about how much he was going to miss her when she left.

'I mean a professional. A… counsellor, or something.'

He sighed. 'I've told you, I don't need to see a shrink.' He placed his hands on her shoulders and tried to look serious. 'What I do need is a quicker route down this bloody incline, because I'm knackered and in desperate need of caffeine.'

She dropped the metal tray onto the snow. 'Then step aboard, good sir, for we shall descend at speed. Today's challenge is called: tray versus snow… although I can't promise a safe landing,' she added, with a shrug.

He stepped over the tray, laughing. 'You're a brave woman, Kate Lawrence.'

She squatted behind him. 'Some might say foolish… Buckle up.'

He rolled his eyes. 'If only. Brace yourself.'

It took all his effort to push them away. It seemed like a lost cause as the tray stuttered over the snow, unwilling to shift. But a sudden drop in the level gave them a jolt of speed, and then next thing he knew, the tray shot off down the slope.

Her scream was so loud, he wasn't sure he'd ever hear properly in his left ear again. Her grip around his middle tightened, as they gained momentum and hurtled down the hill. He suspected a crash landing was likely – something which turned into an inevitability when he saw Suki running towards them.

'Oh, shit!'

His yell did nothing to deter the dog, who sprinted over the snow like an accomplished skier, her tail wagging excitedly as she launched herself into the air and hit them head on. What followed was a series of yelps, swearing and an explosion of snow.

Calvin had no idea how they escaped injury. Amongst the laughter, screaming and plenty of blonde dog hair, all three were thrown into the air, before landing with a thud in the snow.

He couldn't have moved, even if Suki hadn't been standing on his chest, alternating between barking and licking his face, as though he'd invented the best game ever.

'Get off me, you daft dog,' he said, easing her away so he could search for his co-pilot. 'Kate? Are you still alive?'

She struggled to sit up. 'Just about,' she said, spitting snow and wiping it from her face. Her hair was matted, her cheeks were bright pink and she looked slightly dazed. But she surprised him by yelling, 'Hooray! We did it! We won the battle of tray versus snow!' She pinned him with a smile that threatened to melt the snow quicker than if he'd had a blow-torch to hand. 'Tell me that doesn't feel good?'

He couldn't help laughing. Despite the pounding in his head, the ache in his bum and the sadness in his heart at what

the future held for Rose Court, at that precise moment in time
he did indeed feel bloody good.

And the reason was Kate Lawrence.

Chapter Nineteen

Thursday, 23rd December

As Kate escaped the hot kitchen and headed outside to dispose of the waste, she prided herself on having managed to keep occupied for an entire seven hours, without allowing her mind to dwell, which was quite an achievement. Especially as there were any number of thoughts that had the potential to derail her. Spending a further day trapped at Rose Court was one; thinking about Calvin was another. Because however much she tried to ignore it, she liked Calvin. *Really* liked him. And that was why she needed to leave. Staying was causing her fragile heart too much grief. There was only so much baking and present wrapping she could do to occupy her time.

A loud bang from the wooden outbuilding prevented her heading back inside. Concerned an animal might have found its way into the storeroom, she went to investigate, only to stumble across a bizarre scene, similar to a nativity play. Stacked hay bales formed a semicircle, and loose straw had been scattered across the floor.

Even more surprising was the sight of Hanna on her knees, rubbing oil into a wooden crib, and Alex sanding down a piece of wood. 'Goodness, what's going on here?' she said, her eyes growing wide.

'We make festive grotto for Jacob,' Hanna said, her outfit of black leggings and fitted jumper making her look like a spy about to take on Jason Bourne in a martial arts battle.

In contrast, Alex looked like someone from *The Repair Shop*. His leather apron was covered in sawdust and his face was hidden behind a huge pair of goggles. 'Natalie was upset she couldn't take Jacob to see Father Christmas because of the weather,' he said, pointing to a wire coat-hanger dangling from a rafter. 'We're making him a mobile to go above his cot.'

Kate could make out one of the shapes was a sheep. It was very cute. 'I'm sure Natalie will be really touched. Did you make the crib, too?'

'Hanna's quite the carpenter,' Alex said, sounding strangely proud as he watched Hanna rubbing oil on to the slatted wood. 'She's teaching me how to whittle.'

'Right… well, I'm sure it's a skill that will come in handy,' Kate said, even though she wasn't entirely sure what whittling was.

Hanna shook out her cloth. 'In Poland we have culture of making things. Families have no money to buy expensive gifts. We make gifts. A tradition we pass down to each generation. Is good skill to have.'

The care home's head nurse was a woman of many talents, it seemed. 'The crib's beautiful, Hanna. Jacob's a lucky boy.' Kate turned to watch her cousin sanding the wood, showing a level of focus she hadn't seen before. 'You're definitely staying here for Christmas, then?'

Alex nodded. 'Hopefully, I'm staying permanently.'

'How do you mean?'

'This place needs an office manager: someone to run the books, and deal with the finances and admin side of things. I'd like to be that person.'

'But the future of the care home is still undecided,' Kate said, cautiously. 'You do realise that, don't you?'

Alex shrugged. 'There's a possibility Calvin might not sell, and instead decide to stay and manage the place himself. If he does, he'll need an office manager.'

Kate was flummoxed. 'And that's what you want to do? Work here permanently?'

'I like it here, I feel like I fit in. And I like the people,' he said, glancing at Hanna. 'I think it's a job I could be really good at.'

Kate couldn't have been more shocked if her cousin had said he wanted to be a scuba-diving instructor. But what he said made sense – he did look at home here. He socialised with the residents, he helped the staff and he'd done an excellent job dealing with the care-home finances. 'You might be right. But I wouldn't want you to get your hopes up. I'm not sure Calvin has decided anything yet.'

'Why shouldn't I get my hopes up?' he said, sounding unusually assertive. 'Life is what you make it, isn't that what everyone says? You have to fight for what you want and make good things happen. If Calvin knows he has my support and I'm willing to do whatever it takes to help him, it might give him the courage to stay and manage the place himself.'

'Crikey, where has all this positivity come from?' Kate was amazed by the change in her normally morose cousin. 'I've never heard you be so proactive before. It's a lot to get my head around.'

'Someone's been helping me work on my confidence,' he said, with another quick glance at Hanna. 'I need to trust in my abilities more.'

Kate's head went into a spin. Alex had a crush on Hanna? Heavens. This wasn't going to end well. Women like Hanna did not fall for men like Alex – they ate them for breakfast.

But when she looked at Hanna, she couldn't have been more surprised: she was smiling. Well, sort of smiling. The Hanna equivalent of smiling. A neutral expression with a hint of affection. Boudicca was finally thawing… and it seemed her cousin was providing the heat.

'Then I hope it works out for you,' Kate said, smiling at Alex and wondering how she hadn't noticed this fledgling relationship developing before now. Clearly, she hadn't been paying attention – she'd been too focused on her own dramas.

Leaving them to their woodwork, Kate crossed the snowy courtyard towards the main building. If anything, the weather was getting worse: fresh snow had fallen overnight, making the terrain even more treacherous.

As she entered the kitchen, she could hear voices.

'He should've been back ages ago,' Esme said, sounding concerned. 'It'll be dark soon. I'm worried about him.'

Kate stamped her feet on the doormat, dislodging the snow.

'I'm sure he'll be fine,' Geraldine replied, her hands covered in wet dough. 'He's a strong lad. He'd let us know if there was a problem.'

Esme spotted Kate by the door. 'Ah, Kate, darling. Have you heard from Calvin? He walked into the village to collect the turkey from the butcher's and he's not back yet.'

Kate glanced at the kitchen clock. 'What time did he leave?'

'Before lunch. It's been over three hours. He should be back by now.'

Kate removed her apron. 'Have you tried calling him?'

'I can't use those blessed mobile things,' Esme said, dismissing the idea with a hand wave. 'Can you call him for me and check he's okay?'

'Of course.' She wanted to know he was okay, too. It was a long time to be stuck outdoors in such extreme conditions.

Esme and Geraldine watched her as she called him – Esme's expression one of uneasiness, Geraldine's pure intrigue. If the woman was looking for gossip, she was going to be disappointed – unless she ventured outside and stumbled across Hanna and Alex in the shed. But perhaps Geraldine already knew. Maybe Kate was the only one who didn't.

Calvin's phone continued to ring. 'He's not answering.'

'That can't be good.' Esme went over to the window and peered out. 'Do you think someone should go and look for him?'

'Who d'you suggest we send?' Geraldine kneaded a lump of bread dough. 'In case you hadn't noticed, we're not the fittest bunch.'

'Speak for yourself,' Esme said, glaring at Geraldine. 'I'm considered extremely fit for my age.'

Geraldine smirked. 'Are you volunteering for the job?'

'I was thinking of asking Nelson.'

Kate ended the call. 'Nelson's covering for Hanna. Don't worry, I'll go.'

Esme looked hopeful.

Geraldine looked appalled. 'Then we'll have two people missing.'

'But he could be injured,' Esme said, sounding exasperated. 'Lying in a ditch somewhere. Or worse, supposing his heart's given out?' She sagged against the table. 'Oh, God, he's had a heart attack, hasn't he?'

'I'm sure he hasn't,' Kate said, praying he hadn't. 'He's probably in the pub having a beer.'

Esme rubbed her chest. 'Then why isn't he answering his phone?'

'Bad signal?' Kate was clutching at straws, but panicking wouldn't help. 'To be on the safe side, I'll go and look for him.'

Geraldine scoffed. 'What makes you think you'll cope with the conditions any better than him? Supposing you do find him, and he's injured, what then? How are you going to get him home?'

The woman had a point. 'I'll cross that bridge when I come to it. For now, we need to know what's happened to him. The longer we leave it, the darker and colder it's going to get.' She headed for the door. 'I'm going to look for him.'

Rowan almost bumped into her, as he entered the kitchen. 'Look for who?'

Geraldine flicked her tea towel at him when he pinched a mince pie. '*Oi*, those are for tomorrow! Get your mitts off them.'

Rowan took a defiant bite. 'Delicious, darling... Now, who's missing?'

'Calvin.' Esme pushed away from the table. 'He's not back from the village.'

'Oh, that's not good.' Rowan wiped pastry crumbs from his waistcoat. 'Are we hatching a rescue plan?'

Kate tried to sidestep him. 'I'm going to retrace his steps and see if I can find him.'

Rowan caught her arm. 'On foot? Not a good idea, darling.'

'How else am I going to find him? The roads are inaccessible.'

Rowan looked up at the ceiling. 'What's that, Ursula…? Horseback? Excellent idea.' His eyes dipped to Kate's. 'Ursula suggests you travel by horseback.'

'Well, Ursula is not being helpful,' Kate said, trying not to roll her eyes. 'We don't have a horse.'

'Yes, we do.' Rowan disappeared from the kitchen.

Kate turned to Esme and Geraldine. 'Any idea what that's about?'

'Not a clue.' Geraldine banged down her dough. 'Unless he's referring to Bernard.'

Kate looked at Esme, who shrugged and said, 'Don't ask me, I've no idea.'

Fifteen minutes later, Kate wondered if she'd been transported to a parallel universe. One where it was considered normal to be wrapped up like the Michelin Man and perched precariously on top of a stone pillar about to mount a humungous great shire horse called… unsurprisingly, Bernard.

Natalie secured the reins. 'I would offer to go myself, but Jacob's refusing to have his nap and he's grumpy from teething. I don't want to leave him.'

'It's fine, really,' Kate said, faking a confidence she didn't feel. 'It wouldn't be fair to ask you to go anyway.'

'But I'm the one who can ride.' Natalie flipped the reins over the horse's head.

'Kate will be fine!' Rowan yelled from the care-home steps, clutching Esme as they huddled together. 'You said it yourself: Bernard only travels at walking speed, and he knows these lanes backwards.'

Apparently, Bernard was owned by the neighbouring farmer and carried out highly prestigious jobs such as pulling a trap through the village so the farmer's wife could water the hanging baskets.

'Besides, how hard can it be to ride a horse?' Rowan yelled, causing Kate to turn and glare at him.

'I guess I'm about to find out,' she said, steadying herself, ready to mount the blessed thing.

She must be out of her tiny mind to be doing this. If it was anyone other than Calvin, she wouldn't be. But the idea of him being hurt sent pure dread coursing through her. It couldn't be good for his heart condition to be out in this cold.

Leaning forwards, she lifted her leg and hauled herself onto the animal.

It wasn't the most graceful manoeuvre she'd ever performed. Her face was buried in the horse's knotted mane and her bum was poking in the air – although, to be fair, she couldn't imagine Bernard was enjoying the situation any more than she was. One moment he'd been tucked up in his stable, wrapped in a blanket and eating oats, the next he was standing in the freezing cold being mounted by a woman who knew more about nuclear science than she did about horse riding.

She pushed herself upright. 'And you're sure the farmer is okay about us taking him?'

'He was fine,' Natalie said, refusing to make eye contact, which didn't bode well. 'Now, remember what I said about pulling on the reins. Don't tug too hard, he'll know what direction you want him to go. He's an old hand.' She handed Kate the reins. 'Ready?'

Kate drew in a shaky breath. 'As I'll ever be.'

'Good luck!' Esme waved as if Kate was heading off to battle. 'Find my boy!'

Rowan crossed his heart. 'And don't get lost! Those spirits are a ruthless bunch!'

Helpful.

'I'll be fine!' Kate yelled, squeezing her feet like Natalie had demonstrated. 'I'll be back before you know it.' Assuming she didn't freeze to death, get thrown off the horse or get run down by ethereal beings. And to think she'd considered facing bankruptcy a challenge.

With no saddle, Kate had to rely on balance and her inner thigh muscles to keep her upright – attributes not currently included in her CV.

Thankfully, Bernard walked steadily down the driveway and onto the lane with little input from her. The further they travelled, the quieter and darker it became. It was as if the snow had covered the landscape with a giant white blanket, blocking out all noise and movement. It was impossible to see where the lane ended and the woodland began. The trees were so still, it was like they were painted onto the skyline, their bony branches silhouetted against the purple backdrop like splayed fingers.

Despite wearing several layers of clothing, she was freezing. It was like her face had been anaesthetised. She'd lost all feeling in her nose and cheeks, and her teeth rattled comically, like something from a cartoon. But she wasn't about to let her discomfort detract from her mission of finding Calvin.

A sudden noise in the woods startled her. Gripping Bernard's mane, she wondered if she was about to encounter another load of woodland screaming and manic birds threatening to peck her eyes out. But when the noise came again, she realised it was just a fox crying.

As they approached Fright Corner, she searched for the Highwayman's tree, imagining the sight of his body pinned to the trunk, impaled by a sword, but it was impossible see anything when it was covered in snow. Just as well, really. She wasn't sure her nerves could cope with encountering a wayward ghost.

And then she saw it. A shadow in the distance. The outline of a lonesome figure staggering down the middle of the lane. Logic dictated the figure was human and very much alive, but it didn't prevent her mind from fleetingly wondering if it was a ghost. The Highwayman, perhaps? Or the monk, searching for his lost love? It was neither. As the figure drew closer, she realised it was Calvin.

'Oh, thank God,' she said, tugging Bernard to a halt. 'You're not dead, then.'

Calvin stopped walking and stared up at her, as if not quite sure what he was seeing. 'Bloody hell, why are you on a horse?'

'I've come to your rescue,' she said, with a mock salute. 'I appreciate I'm not a gallant knight on a magnificent steed, but a solicitor mounted on a moth-eaten shire horse, but this was all we could come up with at short notice.' She patted the horse's neck. 'No offence, Bernard.'

Calvin blinked up at her. 'Have you been drinking?'

'Not yet – I suspect I will be later. I'll need something to thaw my digits, which are in danger of dropping off.' She smiled down at him, relieved to find him in one piece. He was wearing his familiar thick padded jacket over a hoodie, his baseball cap covering his mass of hair. 'Are you ready to be rescued? In case you haven't noticed, it's pickin' freezing out here.'

He looked confused. 'Why would you think I needed rescuing?'

'You've been gone hours, it's getting dark and you weren't answering your phone. Esme assumed you were lying in a ditch somewhere.'

'Dramatic.' His eye-roll was visible even in the darkness. 'The delivery van was held up due to the bad weather, so the butcher didn't have our order ready. I would've called, but I had no phone signal. I didn't think anyone would miss me yet.'

'Well, they did.' She noticed the thick rope tied around his middle and attached to a wooden crate. 'What's that?'

He glanced behind. 'Makeshift sledge. I had no idea Geraldine had ordered such a huge turkey, as well as joints of beef and gammon, and forty pigs-in-blankets, so carrying it wasn't an option. The butcher gave me this old crate to use. It works, but it's slow going.'

'I can imagine.' She noticed his slumped shoulders. 'You look weary.'

'I am.' He rubbed his face. 'I'm knackered, freezing cold and a bit fed up,' he said, smiling up at her with tired eyes. 'Sorry.'

'Just as well I showed up, then. Think of it as a Christmas miracle.'

He shook his head. 'I still can't believe you're riding a horse. I had no idea you could ride.'

'I can't. This is the result of a crash lesson from Natalie, coupled with praying that Bernard behaves himself. Thankfully, he seems pretty chilled.' She stroked his matted mane. 'Get on, then.'

Calvin's eyes grew wide. 'Can he take our combined weight?'

'According to Natalie. But you'll have to climb up – if I get down, I'll never get on again. I had help getting this far.'

He looked at the crate. 'We'll never get the meat up there as well.'

'Is the rope long enough to drag it behind us?'

'Only one way to find out.' Calvin pulled the crate towards him and stepped on it.

'Before you climb up, can you turn Bernard around so he's facing the right way? I don't fancy attempting a seventeen-point turn with us up here and the meat crate down there. It has disaster written all over it.'

Calvin took the reins and steered Bernard around. 'This is not how I saw this afternoon panning out.'

'No…? Surreal is the new normal in my world.'

He smiled. 'Tell me about it.'

Finally, they were facing the right direction.

She watched him balancing on the crate, before jumping up and landing across Bernard's rump with a grunt.

The horse shifted his weight, as if to say, '*Oi*, mind what you're doing back there!'

The sudden movement sent them both off balance and Kate had to grab the horse's mane to stop herself falling off. 'Sorry, Bernard. We're amateurs. You deserve better, I know.'

'Are you talking to a horse?' Calvin swung his leg over Bernard's back end. 'Christ, this is hard.'

'Now you know why I wanted to stay up here. And I'm not talking to Bernard, so much as acknowledging his discomfort. This can't be fun for him.'

'It's not fun for me, either.' His body bumped against hers as he shifted into position.

Speak for yourself, she thought. This was the closest she'd been to a man in a long while. Well, apart from yesterday's sledging… and their kiss last Sunday, but she was trying not to think about that. Feeling the length of his body against hers was not entirely unpleasant.

Calvin adjusted the rope attached to the crate and snaked an arm around her waist. His face was next to hers, his warm breath tickling her cheek. It was a moment before he seemed to register the intimacy of their position. 'Cosy,' he said, clearing his throat.

'Indeed.' He was shivering and his hands were like ice. 'Let's hope we don't land face down in the snow again.' She felt him smile, and wanted nothing more than to cuddle him and warm him up. Thankfully, any romantic notions involving the two of them galloping off into the twilight were dampened by the sound of Bernard releasing a huge blast of gas. 'Bernard! That's hardly polite.'

Calvin laughed. 'I think it might be payback for us over-loading him.'

'Well, you've made your point,' she said, clicking her heels in an effort to get the horse moving. 'Let's go.'

It took a few attempts to persuade Bernard to move; he seemed to be sulking.

Calvin tugged on the rope as they slowly pulled away, dragging the meat crate behind them. 'So this is the first time you've ridden a horse?'

'Second. The first time didn't go so well.' She lifted her arm. 'Slide your free hand inside my coat. Why didn't you wear gloves?'

'I don't have any,' he said, tucking his hand under her coat. 'So what happened the first time? Did you fall off?'

'Not quite.' She ignored the flutter in her belly when his hand touched her midriff. 'I'd just turned eleven, and Aunty Connie bought me a riding lesson for my birthday. I was plonked on top of a bored-looking pony called Trigger and led around a field for what felt like an eternity, before the instructor unclipped the lead and let me ride solo.'

'What happened?'

'A tree happened.' She felt Calvin's cheek crease against hers. 'I managed to steer the pony towards a giant oak tree, and whereas the horse was able to travel beneath the low-hanging branches, I spent the next ten minutes being smacked in the face by them.'

He laughed.

'The instructor kept yelling at me to change direction, while Alex remained doubled-up on the fence, laughing his head off.'

Calvin hugged her tighter. 'Were you hurt?'

'No, but I spent the next twenty-four hours sneezing from all the tree pollen up my nose. It was not a good experience.'

'Poor Katiekins,' he whispered, sending a shiver up her spine. 'Thank you for overcoming such a traumatic experience to come to my rescue.'

'Are you taking the piss?'

'I wouldn't dream of it.'

'Then why are you laughing?'

'Because if anyone had told me a year ago that this is what I'd be doing right now, I'd have assumed they were on something. Like you said, it's beyond surreal.'

'Which bit?'

'All of it. The weather, the horse… you. My life is unrecognisable.' He sounded bemused. 'I'm just puzzled as to why I'm not more disturbed by it.'

'Well… give it time,' she said, her shivering masking the shake in her legs. 'This isn't over yet. I still have Rowan's voice in my head, warning me about the phantom coach and horses that reputedly haunt this section of road. If rumours are to be believed, we could be mowed down at any moment.'

'I'll make a bet with you. If we encounter a spectral carriage between now and returning to Rose Court, I will personally pay for you to go on a round-the-world cruise, stopping at any destination of your choice.'

She twisted her head to look at him. 'Why a cruise?'

'You said you envied your aunty heading off on a cruise. I thought it might be something you'd enjoy.'

She focused ahead, in case her expression gave her away. Why did he have to be so darned nice? 'One flaw.'

'Which is?'

'I can't go on a cruise if I'm dead.' She steered Bernard towards the lane leading up to Rose Court. 'If we encounter the phantom coach then we're done for. Haven't you heard the saying, "dying of fright"? It's not used without good reason.'

He rested his chin on her shoulder. 'Nobody's dying tonight.'

'Well... good.' She glanced away from the sight of his dimples. Up close, they were even more lethal. 'But then I'll have lost the bet.'

'Then you'll have to pay up.'

'I might've known there'd be a catch.' She rolled her eyes. Not that he could see, but still. 'What's my forfeit?'

'Staying at Rose Court for Christmas.'

This statement should have caused more displeasure than it did, but the idea of staying at Rose Court did make her feel a little excited. It wasn't like she wanted to leave; it was just in her best interests to do so. 'That's a loaded bet.'

'That's why I made it.' His voice was barely a whisper. 'I want you to stay.'

The gargoyles perched on the pillars viewed her with disdain, as if they were as disgusted with her as she was. It wasn't like she hadn't tried to escape. The weather had conspired against her. She wasn't staying for any other reason... but she knew that was a lie.

'Doesn't look like I'm going to be able to leave anyway,' she said, as Rose Court loomed ahead. 'More snow is due and it's Christmas Eve tomorrow. I might've missed my last chance.'

'Then we're both winners.'

She glanced over her shoulder. 'How do you figure that?'

His eyes met hers. 'We don't die of fright... and you get to stay. I'd call that a win.'

His tender expression turned her stomach to pulp, and she knew it was a lost cause. She'd only gone and fallen in love with Calvin bloody Johnson, hadn't she?

What an absolute fool.

'Oh, look,' he said, drawing her attention to the front of the care home. 'The welcome committee have come out to greet us. Lucky us.'

Lucky, indeed.

Chapter Twenty

Christmas Eve

The landscape surrounding the care home had finally started to thaw. The rigid icicles hanging from the rafters had begun to melt and the sheets of ice making the driveway precarious had dissolved into the gravel below. Instead of a harsh winter's scene, the view from the staff room now resembled something from a picturesque Christmas card.

Leaning against the window frame, Calvin cuddled Jacob closer, glad of the comfort of another body pressed against his – even a tiny one. He'd grown accustomed to these views. He still missed city life, but he'd adjusted to country living. He enjoyed his early morning runs with Suki, being able to breathe in clean air, with no hint of car fumes, and savour the sound of birdsong. Country life might not be enough on its own to keep him stimulated, but with Ashford only a train stop away, with its shops, restaurants, bars and sports facilities, the area had more to offer than he'd first imagined.

It wasn't just the area he'd become attached to – something that had become apparent when he'd arrived back at the care home yesterday, having been 'rescued' by Kate. The image of her appearing through the snowy haze perched on a giant shire horse had been the most surreal, funny and touching moment of his entire life. He couldn't imagine Ainsley ever coming to his rescue like that. The idea that someone cared about him that much was... astonishing. And touching. And very confusing.

And it wasn't just Kate who had been concerned. They'd been welcomed home as if returning from a dangerous arctic mission, wrapped in thick blankets, given hot chocolate – laced with whisky – and bundled into the lounge and instructed to warm themselves by the fire.

It didn't matter that he was a grown man capable of taking care of himself, or that his 'carers' were four decades older than him and in need of care themselves. They'd insisted on ensuring he was okay – Kate, too.

The pampering hadn't let up all evening. Geraldine fed them casserole, Larry serenaded them with Christmas classics, Esme and Rowan plied them with 'medicinal' drinks, and Hanna insisted on checking his vitals. He'd been too dulled by whisky shots to object.

The evening ended with them lazing around the lounge, watching *Home Alone* – Kate's idea – and drifting into a contented sleep, like some weird hippy commune. Strangely, he hadn't hated it. It had felt normal. Like this was how his life was meant to be. And if that wasn't completely absurd, he didn't know what was. Maybe he did need professional help after all.

The staff-room door opened and Nelson appeared, wearing his blue nurse's tunic, and flopped onto the couch. 'You on babysitting duties?'

Calvin smiled at his charge. Jacob was wrapped in a cosy onesie, ready for his outdoor adventure. 'Just while Natalie gets changed. We're off to see Father Christmas.'

Nelson let out a huge yawn. 'Ah, the infamous nativity scene. No one can accuse this place of not going the extra mile.'

'Tired?'

'I blame that gigantic lunch,' he said, rubbing his stomach. 'I've never eaten so much in my life – I'm stuffed.' Another yawn escaped him. 'Kate's in with Deshad and Priya, giving them advice about wills, so I thought I'd grab five minutes.'

Calvin adjusted his grip on Jacob. 'You want us to leave and give you some peace?'

'You're fine. I'm happy relaxing for a moment.' Nelson noticed the document lying on the coffee table. 'You been checking out care-home qualifications?'

Calvin nodded. 'I started looking at football training courses, but ended up researching care home management instead.'

'Did you discover anything interesting?'

'That I'm more qualified to coach football than I am to look after care residents,' he said, trying not to sound despondent. It was beyond depressing to discover how little he was qualified to do, other than play football. 'I thought there might be a fast-track route into care management, but it takes years to reach the required level.'

Nelson raised his eyebrows. 'You don't need formal qualifications to manage a care home, mate.'

'But it's recommended.' He moved away from the window. 'The website says you need a degree in social work, a nursing diploma or an equivalent NVQ qualification in health and social care. I don't even have A levels,' he said, ashamed by his lack of education.

Nelson flicked through the document. 'There's the option of taking a management route.'

'I don't have any management training either.'

'It says here you need strong leadership skills, strategic thinking, project and organisational management, and good communication.' He looked up. 'Mate, you have these in spades.'

'I doubt the local authority would agree with you, or any family looking to place a loved one. They're not going to be impressed by someone running a home without proper training.'

Nelson slid the document onto the table. 'But it doesn't fall to you to provide all that. You need to build a team around you with the relevant training to support the skills you already have. Once the probate money comes through, you can hire people with specialist social care training. You don't have to be an expert yourself. You just need to know what's needed and how to manage the place – which you already do, and on severely depleted resources.' He stretched out his arms. 'Seriously, mate, don't underestimate your skills.'

Calvin shrugged. 'Maybe.'

'You don't believe me?' Nelson rested a hand on his shaved head. 'If you offered me a full-time job here, I'd jump at it.'

Calvin blinked, surprised. 'Really?'

'Sure. Care work is a thankless task. It's hard work, long hours, exhausting and frustrating. I switched to locum work because it avoids the red tape and restrictions that come with working permanently somewhere. But it's different here. You've created a unique vibe, professional without the bureaucracy. It's cool. Like being part of one big dysfunctional family. I think I fit right in.'

Nelson did fit in. The residents loved him, and even Hanna had given her approval. 'You'd seriously accept a job here?'

'Just say the word.'

Natalie appeared in the doorway, wrapped in her coat. She skipped over to her son, her arms outstretched. 'Ready to meet Father Christmas?' she said, in a sing-song voice. 'Thanks for looking after him, Calvin. Has he been good?'

'An angel.' Calvin handed Jacob over, already missing his warmth.

When Natalie smiled, he noticed that her eyes were no longer rimmed with dark circles. She was looking so much better since Nelson had joined the team. Like a weight had been lifted. 'Are you coming with us?'

'Wouldn't miss it,' he said, looking at Nelson. 'Thanks for the advice, mate. Enjoy your nap.'

'No worries.' Nelson waved a hand. 'Enjoy meeting the big guy.'

Calvin followed Natalie and Jacob downstairs, trying to make sense of his struggles. A year ago everything had been on track and he'd been excited about the next stage of his life. Marriage, kids and, with any luck, another ten years playing football. He'd never imagined what his life might look like post-football. Even if he had, he'd never have envisaged spending it alone. The idea of not having a family depressed him almost as much as the loss of his career.

He realised there were no easy decisions. Either way, he was facing uncertainty, whether he stayed in Kent or returned to Leeds.

It was quiet when they arrived downstairs, since everyone was already congregated in the outbuilding. As they left the warmth of the kitchen and crossed the snowy courtyard, they were met by Hanna and Alex, holding lanterns aloft. The entranceway was decorated with twinkling fairy lights, flickering in the dusky light.

'Welcome to Santa's grotto,' Alex said, bowing.

Hanna looked down at Jacob. 'Have you been good boy?' she asked, not quite managing to hide the accusation in her voice. 'Only good children get to meet the *gwiazdor*.'

Jacob gurgled and kicked his tiny legs, making Natalie laugh. 'Yes, I think so, too, Jacob.'

Hanna stood back to allow them inside. 'Then you may enter.'

The sight that greeted them made Calvin laugh. It wasn't the cute nativity crib scene that tickled him, or the array of candles balancing on hay bales – which, as health and safety officer, he shouldn't approve of – it was the cast of characters waiting to perform that cracked him up.

Geraldine, Esme and Rowan were dressed as the three wise men, complete with tea-towel head coverings, wooden staffs and dressing gowns tied around their middles with what looked like the curtain tie-backs from the library. They stood in a semicircle, trying to look wise and seriously failing.

In the far corner, seated on a hay bale, was Father Christmas. Not any old Santa: this was the coolest Saint Nicholas that Calvin had ever seen. Lucky Larry was wearing a dark-red lounge suit, a makeshift white beard made from cotton wool and his velvet green Santa hat perched on his head. With Rowan's emerald green cravat tied around his neck, complete with matching handkerchief tucked in his pocket, he looked quite debonair.

Calvin leant against the door frame, smiling as the three wise men launched into 'We Three Kings', and Natalie carried Jacob over to meet Father Christmas.

Behind him, the barn door opened and a draught blew through as Kate appeared, minus her coat. She was wearing a dark green sparkly dress that was too big for her, on loan from his grandmother, and tights embroidered with mistletoe. Rubbing her arms, she grinned as she took in the scene ahead. 'Cute.'

He lifted his arm, offering her the chance to get closer and warm up. 'Cold?'

'A bit.' She slid in next to him. 'I didn't want to miss this.'

He pulled her close and rubbed her shoulder, feeling her shiver against him. He was relieved that the awkwardness of earlier in the week had disappeared. They were back to being mates again, even if that did bring with it a different set of challenges.

Physically, it was a no-brainer. He liked being with her, he was attracted to her and cuddling her felt totally right – like it was the most natural thing in the world.

It was only when his mind began to question his motives that complications arose. He had no idea where he was going to be living, he was undecided about his career and he was still healing from a broken heart. How could he offer her anything when he was so uncertain about his future? She deserved better than that. She'd been messed around enough. He'd hate himself if he added to her hurt – even though the idea of never seeing her again made him feel physically sick.

He rested his cheek against her soft hair. 'Nelson was falling asleep when I left him. Did you have to wake him?'

'Deshad said not to bother,' she said, humming along to the singing. 'Priya was drifting off herself when I left, so there was nothing that needed doing.'

He was glad Nelson could catch up on some sleep – he'd been working as hard as everyone else these last few days.

He wondered if the man had been serious about wanting a permanent position at Rose Court. It was a compliment, if nothing else. Nelson was an exceptional nurse. He was also proving to be a good mate.

Calvin's attention returned to the sight of Jacob being cradled in Lucky Larry's arms. It made him wistful for a family of his own. 'I hear you've been helping Deshad and Priya with a will?'

'I've drafted something for Deshad, but Priya doesn't have the capacity to make decisions, sadly. At least he has power of attorney for her, so that's something.'

'Can he afford to have a will drawn up? I know money's tight.'

She glanced up, her blue eyes dilated in the dim candlelight. 'We agreed payment of a different kind,' she said, keeping her voice low. Not that they could be heard over the gusto of the three wise men singing. 'It's a drawing of the view from their window, looking out over the care-home grounds. Deshad thought I might like it as a reminder of my time here.'

'I didn't know Deshad liked drawing?' Calvin was surprised. 'Maybe I should get him a proper art kit. I worry about him being stuck in that room all day. I'd feel better if he had a hobby to keep him occupied.'

Kate's face broke into a smile. 'Look at you, advocating the benefits of having a hobby.'

He rolled his eyes. 'Maybe I'm evolving.'

'Maybe you are.' She turned back to the nativity scene, smiling.

The three wise men switched to singing 'Little Donkey', as Larry carried baby Jacob over to the crib to show him his present.

Calvin nodded to where Jacob was reaching out to touch the mobile dangling above the crib, his eyes wide and mesmerised. 'You holding up okay?'

She gave a little shrug. 'It's not as if the sight of a cute baby meeting Father Christmas is touching. So what if there's

253

candlelight, singing and fairy lights. It's not like a trigger, or anything.'

A beat passed, before he spoke. 'Are you crying?'

'Absolutely. You?'

'Bloody close.' When she laughed, he whispered in her ear. 'Shall we escape?'

Her eyes slid up to meet his. 'Yes, please.'

He could argue that it was the emotion of watching Jacob being cute that threatened to undo him, or the ambience of festive music, flickering candlelight and the sight of his grandmother dressed as a biblical king. But in truth, it was holding Kate and feeling her body pressed against his that was causing his mind to short-circuit. For someone determined not to let anything happen between them, he was doing a lousy job.

Leaving the outbuilding, they crossed the snow-covered courtyard, shivering and laughing as they slipped on the melting ice.

As they entered the kitchen, they were hit by a wave of heat from the Aga. The scent of mulling spices filled the air, accompanied by the radio playing choral Christmas music.

Trays of mince pies were lined along the table, next to a chocolate log with a snowman perched on top. Geraldine had been busy. Sausage rolls were cooling on the side, along with a selection of cheeses still in their wrappers.

Calvin stamped on the doormat, dislodging the loose snow. 'How Geraldine expects us to eat again after such a huge lunch, I've no idea.'

'It's Christmas,' Kate said, pinching a sausage roll. 'It doesn't matter how much you eat – you can always find room for more.' She took a bite of sausage roll, her hand coming up to catch the flakes.

'Until you can't.' He dragged his gaze away from her mouth, as she licked her fingers.

'At which point you either stop, pass out or throw up, vowing never to eat another thing.' She smiled at him. 'Until the next morning, when it starts all over again.'

'Just as well it's only once a year.'

'True.' Having wiped her hands, she headed out of the kitchen and into the lobby.

He followed her into the library. The room was chilly and the windows were drenched in condensation. The fire hadn't been lit today, and it didn't take long for the temperature to drop in such an old building.

'Here's the drawing I was telling you about,' she said, handing it to him. 'Talented, isn't he?'

Calvin looked at the sketch, amazed at how much detail Deshad had managed to capture. The image was instantly recognisable, a faithful recreation of the view from the couple's bedroom window. But as beautiful as it was, it also made him feel sad – as if the artist was yearning for something he couldn't have. A life outside of the care home, probably. Priya wasn't the only one trapped by her poor health.

He became aware of Kate looking over his shoulder. She smelt faintly of candle wax and warm pastry. 'I'm going to have it framed and put up in my office,' she said, heading over to the window. 'Wherever that might be.'

Her watched her move, missing her close proximity. 'Any luck with the job hunting?'

She kicked off her Ugg boots and climbed onto the window seat. 'I've been offered an interview next week at a firm in Richmond, so I guess that's something. Big firm, good salary, decent benefits. I'd be crazy not to go for it.'

'You don't sound enthusiastic.'

She stretched up on tiptoe and pulled the curtains, and the movement directed his gaze down to her calf muscles, no longer hidden under thick leggings, but shapely in her festive tights. 'Beggars can't be choosers, right?' She climbed off the window seat and rubbed her arms. 'It's cold in here.'

He went over to the fireplace. 'Is it the job you have doubts about, or job-hunting in general?'

She joined him by the fireplace and knelt next to him, watching as he loaded the grate with logs. 'I think it's the idea

255

of working for someone else that's unsettling me. I've enjoyed being my own boss these last couple of months. I know that, technically, I was working for you, but it was nice to manage the case myself and not have to provide updates to a board of directors.' She handed him the fire tongs. 'Do you need these?'

'I will do,' he said, adding kindling to the log pile.

'And then there's the whole mental health issue.'

He stopped loading the fire and looked at her. 'I thought you were feeling better? Your panic attacks seem to have stopped. Or have you just been hiding them from me?'

'No, they've stopped,' she said, unwrapping a box of fire-lighters. 'Or they appear to have. I'm definitely feeling a lot better, and knowing I'll be able to pay off my debts soon is a huge relief.'

'Your ex-husband's debts, you mean.' His fingers brushed hers as she handed him the firelighters. 'You're not to blame, remember?'

'You're right. Let me rephrase… my pathetic excuse of an ex-husband's debts.'

He smiled. 'Better.'

Using his shoulder to lean on, she got up and went over to the desk. 'I'm not foolish enough to believe I'm completely cured, or that certain situations won't act as a trigger, but I'm more worried about coping with the general stress of it all. Long hours, targets, heavy caseloads.' She returned with the lighter and handed it to him. 'Am I up to it?'

'Only you can answer that. But for what it's worth, you're the most resilient person I know. You never cease to amaze me. Not every woman would attempt sledging, or venture into the night on horseback to rescue someone. And it's not like this has been an easy case, but you've handled it well.'

'You mean, apart from yelling at ghosts, accusing the stepladders of trying to topple me off and conversing with portraits of your dead ancestors?'

He grinned, remembering the incident well. 'Apart from that.'

'I'm a walking advert for the deranged, I know.' She held her hands in front of the fire as the flames took hold. 'But you're right, this has been the most challenging case I've ever worked on, and yet it's been the most rewarding. Maybe it's the location. Or the building… It might even be the people,' she said, shooting him a glance. 'But I've loved working here. It's given me a glimpse of the life I want moving forwards. One day I want to be my own boss and take charge of my own destiny.'

He turned to her. 'Self-employed, you mean?'

She nodded. 'I got the idea the other day when I was Christmas shopping. There's a law clinic in Ashford that hires out offices to self-employed solicitors. I had no idea it was even a thing, but now I know it exists, I can't stop thinking about it.' Her loose hair trailed across the side of her face and he wanted to tuck it behind her ear. 'It's wishful thinking, I know.'

'Why is it?'

'I have no home, remember? And no savings. Building a business from scratch takes time. Clients aren't going to come flooding in the moment I announce I'm going solo. I'll need to grow my reputation and client base over time. It requires more planning.' She stared into the fire, her expression thoughtful. 'Maybe one day I'll achieve my dream. In the meantime, I need to find myself a decently paid job and just hope my fragile nerves can cope with the anxiety.' She let out a sigh. 'What other option do I have?'

He prodded the fire with the tongs. 'Does the job have to be in London? You said you liked living here in Kent.'

'I do, but most of the jobs being advertised are in the big cities. I'm trying to be flexible and not discount anywhere because of location.'

He hung the tongs on their stand. 'Won't you be lonely, living somewhere new by yourself?'

She shrugged. 'Probably. Such is life. Hopefully, it won't be forever.'

He hated the idea of her being unhappy, or stressed, in a new job. She deserved so much more than life had thrown at her. He wished he could make it better, but he couldn't sort out his own job situation, let alone resolve someone else's.

He got up and went over to the desk to return the lighter, noticing a pile of small envelopes lying on top. 'I hate to break it to you, but you've missed the last post.'

She strained to see. 'Oh, those aren't for posting,' she said, getting up and coming over. 'Well, not externally, anyway. They're for the game I made.'

'Game?' He skimmed through the envelopes, reading the words written on the front in Kate's neat handwriting. 'Booby Dingle… Spankers Hill Wood… Tickle Cock Bridge… The Blind Fiddler?' He raised an eyebrow. 'What kind of game are you planning here?'

'Not that kind of game,' she said, sloshing him. 'The post-office game.' When he still didn't react, she pointed at the envelopes. 'You said you liked playing it when you were young.'

His face was starting to grow warm. He had a feeling it wasn't down to the fire.

'These are all real places,' she said, nodding at the envelopes. 'I looked them up online. It's amazing what comes up in the search results when you type in unusual place names.' She pointed to a small red postbox sitting on one of the bookcases. 'I made the postboxes out of cardboard. Thankfully, Geraldine had a stash of red tissue paper, and Deshad helped me to cut the letterbox holes. There are thirty of them in total scattered around the ground floor of the building… although I promise there are none hidden in the washing machine. I wouldn't be that cruel,' she said, laughing. But then her smile faded. 'Oh, God, why are you looking at me like that? Have I done something wrong?'

He was struggling to speak. 'You went to all this effort… for me?'

'Well, of course. You're not getting to spend Christmas with your family, so I thought playing a game might make you… I

258

dunno, smile a bit? Nothing like a bit of nostalgia at Christmas-time.' Her unsure gaze was fixed on his. 'Do you… do you like it?'

Like it? He bloody loved it.

More worryingly, he loved *her*.

And that was a much bigger problem than all his other problems added together.

Chapter Twenty-One

Christmas Day

It was gone seven p.m. by the time all the day's festivities had concluded and everything had been tidied away. As worn-out bodies emerged from late afternoon naps and wine glasses were refilled, ready for the evening's entertainment, the group slowly drifted into the lounge, ready to exchange gifts.

Kate relaxed against the sofa cushions, her eyes sleepy from gazing at the flickering Christmas tree lights, as she listened to Larry playing a jazz version of 'If I Didn't Care' on the piano. Was the man a mind reader?

She could vaguely see her sprawled-out reflection in the gilded mirror above the fireplace, the faint sparkle in her blue chiffon top glittering under the candlelight. She'd made an effort with her appearance today, adding silver hoop earrings and wearing a dash of make-up. And although the glow in her cheeks was enhanced from the amount of champagne she'd consumed during lunch, her snowmen slippers ruined any attempts to look classy. But with limited access to anything fancier, it was the best she could do.

At least her clothes fitted today. Unlike yesterday, when she'd spent the entire duration of the post-office game trying not to tread on the hem of Esme's dress as she'd raced around the building in an attempt to referee the game. Who knew octogenarians could be so unscrupulous when it came to competition?

The memory made her smile. The game had proved popular, and everyone had joined in, manically rushing around in search of the postboxes so they could post their letters. As the alcohol consumption had increased, so had the level of cheating. After two hours of laughter, sabotage, and Rowan accusing Ursula of 'hexing' the postboxes, the game was concluded, with Alex and Hanna declared the winners.

Exhausted from the exertion, everyone had collapsed onto the sofas in the lounge and sleepily watched the latest James Bond movie.

Kate had ended up next to Calvin, which had been a blessing and a curse. She wasn't sure how her hand had ended up in his, or when his arm had slid around her, but as she'd rested her head against his shoulder and felt his thumb circling her wrist, she'd felt something shift inside her, like a knot unravelling, leaving her feeling boneless and contented.

Alex suddenly flopped down next to her, dislodging a cushion. 'Have you spoken to the family yet?' He handed her a flute of champagne. Like she needed any more.

'I had a lovely chat with Mum and Brian first thing, and I've just finished FaceTiming your sisters. They said you haven't called them yet.'

'I'll call them later. How were they?'

'Good.' She took a sip of champagne, the bubbles tickling her nose. 'Poor Matt and Zac couldn't get a word in. Megan is annoyed she can't drink this Christmas, and Beth looked like she was hiding a secret, so I expect an announcement later.'

Alex's eyebrows raised. 'You think Matt proposed?'

'Knowing Beth, it was probably the other way around.' She raised her champagne flute. 'Good for her, I say. She deserves to be happy.'

Alex rubbed the back of his neck. 'Talking of which…'

Kate smiled. 'You and Hanna?'

He looked sheepish. 'That obvious?'

'Apparently. Although it seems I was a bit slow on the uptake. Sorry about that, I've been a bit preoccupied of late.'

'I'm the one who should apologise.'

'What for?'

'Neglecting you.' He fiddled with the buttons on his new shirt. She was still getting used to this version of Alex, with his smart haircut and ironed clothes. 'I promised the family I'd look after you during your time here, but I don't think I did a very good job. I kind of got distracted.'

She patted his knee. 'For the nicest of reasons.'

'But it wasn't very cool of me. Sorry.'

'No harm done.' She gave a little shrug. 'I'm fine.'

'Are you?'

She realised he was genuinely worried about her. 'I think so. I'm certainly better than I was. My anxiety levels have lowered, and I'm feeling more positive about the future. I'll be debt-free soon, so onwards and upwards, as they say.'

He nodded slowly. 'But you're still leaving?'

'No reason for me to stay.'

She could feel him looking at her. 'Isn't there?'

How was she supposed to answer that? If things were different... if she was settled in a job and had financial security and Calvin was in the same position, then what? She'd stay? Would it really make a difference? Calvin was drawn to her because he was bruised and needed comfort. She was a temporary fix. Would she still be who he wanted if he was in a better place? No. And she wasn't foolish enough to think otherwise. Calvin was a fantasy. A secret crush. The guy she wanted but couldn't have.

Sighing, she turned to her cousin. 'Have you spoken to Calvin yet about his plans?'

Alex shook his head. 'He's still undecided about what to do, so I don't want to add to his stress. Hanna said he's promised to make a decision before New Year.'

'Well, that's something. I'll keep my fingers crossed everything works out for you.' She reached over and kissed his cheek. 'You deserve to be happy.'

'You do, too.' He squeezed her shoulder and got up to join Hanna, who was playing with Jacob on the floor.

Kate would miss Alex when she left tomorrow. It had been nice working together. He'd found his future here, and she couldn't be happier for him.

Looking around the room, she realised he wasn't the only person she'd miss. Rowan with his ghost stories, Esme and Geraldine with their fussing over her, Natalie's friendship, and Larry's love of music. She'd even miss spending time with Deshad and Priya, despite the sadness of their situation. They needed all the friendship they could get.

And then there was Calvin…

As her eyes searched for him, they landed on Larry instead and he beckoned her over.

Glad of the distraction, she got up and joined him. The last thing she needed was to start dwelling over Calvin and feeling morose. It was Christmas Day, for crying out loud. She should be celebrating.

Larry patted the piano seat next to him. 'Join me in a duet?'

Kate's insides tightened. The idea of performing in public still unnerved her.

He must have sensed her trepidation, because he gave her a nudge. 'It's not like you're playing to a hostile crowd. They're not even sober… and most of them are deaf.'

Kate laughed. 'When you put it like that.'

'Good girl. Your choice.'

It didn't take much thinking about. '"The Man with the Bag". Ella Fitzgerald.'

'Nice.' He ran his nimble fingers effortlessly over the keys, giving her a lengthy introduction. 'Want me to sing?'

'Yes, please.' She settled into position.

There was no way Kate would have played solo, but with Larry's expertise adding intricate runs and enhancing her basic chords, her confidence grew, and by the time they hit the first chorus, she'd relaxed enough to enjoy herself.

Everyone in the room had stopped chatting and were either swaying along to the song or, in Geraldine's case, full-on

263

dancing. Esme and Rowan came over to the piano to join in with the singing.

She risked a glance at Calvin, who had just returned from the cellar with more wine. The expression on his face almost derailed her ability to play. He looked at her with a mixture of pride, happiness and absolute tenderness, and when he unleashed the dimples, she had to look away.

They finished with a big flurry, Larry's voice smooth as chocolate, yet raspy as vintage whisky. There was something incredibly satisfying about receiving rapturous applause and calls for an encore. But one song was enough. Maybe later, when she'd had a few more glasses of bubbly.

Thanking Larry with a kiss, she notched up the experience to another step on her road to recovery. Performing in public was definite progress. However small the audience.

Once the novelty of her playing had subsided, she was glad when Natalie suggested exchanging gifts. It would be Jacob's bedtime soon, and although he'd opened his huge pile of gifts that morning, she wanted him to watch the adults opening theirs.

Kate was happy to hand out the gifts with Calvin, smiling as everyone tried to guess what was inside by squeezing the packages.

At one point, they both reached for the same present and their hands touched. He caught her arm before she could move away, and whispered, 'Well done for playing. You were amazing,' which sent a shiver racing through her.

Feeling stupidly buoyed, she settled down on a beanbag to watch everyone open their presents. When she'd taken part in Secret Santa at work, people rarely put any thought into it, and she'd lost count of the number of wine bottles she'd received. But here everyone had carefully selected something that suited the person.

Geraldine had bought Natalie a voucher for a spa day. In return, Natalie had given the chef a funky neon-pink walking stick. Rowan had purchased theatre tickets for Esme, and she'd got him a 'Haunted House' experience. Larry had bought Deshad noise-cancelling headphones, so he could listen to music without disturbing Priya – which made Deshad cry – and Deshad had given Larry a pencil drawing of one of his framed Motown discs, which made him cry, too.

The funniest exchange involved Hanna and Alex. The head nurse gave him a tool belt, complete with chisels and spirit level, for his excursions into the world of whittling. In return, Alex had bought Hanna a snake..

It was hard to describe the collective reaction as Hanna pulled away the wrapping to reveal a large cage filled with straw, a water bottle and the carcass of a dead mouse.

Amongst the gasps, shock and laughter, Natalie hastily removed Jacob from the floor, and Larry climbed onto the piano stool.

A stunned Hanna stared at the snake for a full minute, before turning to Alex. 'You buy me snake?'

The room held its breath.

Alex nodded slowly. 'It's a royal python. Do you like it?'

She grabbed his face and kissed him.

Kate took this to mean Hanna liked it.

The sight of Hanna and Alex kissing caused further gasps, shock and laughter, followed by raucous clapping and shouts of, 'About bloody time!'

It took a while for the excitement to settle, not least because Suki had taken an instant dislike to the snake, and a heated debate followed about where the creature should live. It was eventually agreed that the wooden outbuilding would be the safest place… for everyone.

Which just left Kate and Calvin to exchange their gifts. Something Kate would have preferred to do without an audience, especially as her budget had been tight and everyone else had been so generous, but there was no escaping it. She just hoped she hadn't misjudged it.

'It's only a bit of fun,' she said, as she handed him the box. 'I hope you like it.'

'I know I will,' he said, tearing off the wrapping. 'It's from you.'

He hadn't spoken loudly, but a few people heard anyway and sighed.

Just as Hanna had done when faced with the snake, Calvin stared at his present with a look of shock. Thankfully, the silence didn't last quite so long, and a beat later, his eyes drifted to hers. 'You bought me Pop-Up Pirate?'

'It's silly, I know,' she said, feeling self-conscious with everyone watching her. 'It was meant to be a bit of fun.'

'It's… perfect.' His face broke into the most adorable grin.

Esme sniffed and reached for a tissue. 'You sulked for days when that game got broken. You were heartbroken.'

Calvin rolled his eyes. 'Yeah, thanks, *Granny*.'

Esme threw a cushion at him. 'Less of the granny talk, thank you.'

Calvin returned the game to its box and got to his feet. 'Ready for your present?'

'I guess.' Kate couldn't imagine what he might have bought her. Supposing it was a bottle of wine? She wasn't sure she could cope with that.

It wasn't wine. When the huge parcel appeared from behind the piano, she felt her eyes grow wide. 'What on earth is that?' she said, stunned by the size of the thing.

He carried it over and placed it carefully in front of her. 'Open it and find out.'

Her hands began to shake as she tore away the sheets of wrapping. Beneath were layers of bubble wrap, disguising the shape. But the moment she saw the black leather casing, silver clasps and long slender neck, she knew what it was.

'You got me a guitar?'

'It's that, or a tommy gun,' Larry said, laughing.

She was almost too overwhelmed to open it. The shake in her hands didn't let up as she released the clasps and lifted the lid. Inside was an acoustic Fender Classic, like her dad's. Mahogany, with a darker base.

'I hope it's okay?' Calvin sounded uncertain.

There were a number of things Kate avoided doing in public. Crying was definitely one of them. Shakily getting to her feet, she swallowed hard, blinking rapidly, and tried to escape the onslaught she knew was coming. 'Excuse me a moment,' she said, running from the room.

Ignoring his calls, she continued running. She had to. She wasn't sure whether she was about to have a panic attack or throw up. Either way, she didn't want an audience.

As her breaths grew shorter, her running slowed and she was dizzy by the time she'd climbed two flights of stairs to the second floor. Tears streamed down her face as she staggered down the hallway, gulping in air and feeling her chest tighten.

By the time she reached her room, she felt close to passing out.

She made it into the bathroom, before slumping against the closed door and sliding to the floor.

Closing her eyes, she rested her forehead on her arms, trying to calm her breathing.

It wasn't long before the inevitable. A knock on the bathroom door.

She hadn't expected anything less, even if she had hoped for longer to compose herself.

'Kate? Are you okay?' He sounded distraught, and she couldn't blame him.

'I'm so sorry,' she managed to say. 'I just wasn't expecting that.'

'Was it too much? It was too much, wasn't it? Oh, God, Kate, I'm sorry. I didn't mean to upset you. I just wanted to thank you for everything you've done.'

'It's fine, really.' She wiped at her eyes, feeling foolish.

'It's not fine. Are you having a panic attack?'

'I don't think so.'

'Are you sure? Can I come in?'

'Just give me a moment.'

'Okay, but I'm not leaving. I'm staying right here.'

She rested her head against the door and closed her eyes, her mind tumbling with an array of thoughts and images, flickering in and out. Photos of her dad playing his guitar. Her learning to play it as a child. The grief and anger she'd felt when Tristan had sold it.

All the loss she'd experienced over the last few years came tumbling back, unleashed and raw, triggered by an act of kindness. A man who had only been in her life a short time, but who had shown her endless support and friendship, and had cared enough to buy her a replacement guitar, knowing how much it would mean to her.

'I'm sorry I ran off,' she said, knowing she owed him an explanation. 'Please don't think it's because I don't love the gift, I do. It's just…' She hesitated, but there was no avoiding the truth. 'You see… well, it's just that my dad took his own life.'

A deathly silence followed. She could almost feel the weight of it seeping through the closed door. When he did speak, his voice was barely a whisper. 'Shit. I'm so sorry, Kate.'

'It's okay, you didn't know. How could you? I never told you.'

More silence followed. She could almost imagine his mind whirring as he took in the enormity of what she'd said. 'I should've realised getting a guitar would remind you of your dad. It was thoughtless of me.'

'Are you kidding me? It was incredibly kind of you. You just caught me unaware, that's all.' She wiped her damp cheeks. 'It's a lovely gift and I'll treasure it always.'

It was a while before Calvin spoke. 'Why did he take his own life? Do you know?'

'That's the million-dollar question. I guess we'll never know for certain.'

'Had he been depressed?'

'Who knows. Although Mum said he'd been unusually quiet and preoccupied in the weeks leading up to it. He was stressed about work, and he'd drunkenly confessed to a mate that he was scared of letting his family down. He worried about not being a good provider, and being more of a burden than a help.'

'That must've been difficult for your mum.'

'It tortured her for years. They'd had their difficulties, but she never dreamt he felt that way. It made her incredibly angry that he never confided in her.'

'I can imagine.'

She tore off a wodge of loo roll and wiped her eyes. 'Maybe if he had, she could've reassured him everything was okay. Or at least persuaded him to get some help. But mental health wasn't talked about so much in those days. It's hard enough talking about it now, as we both know.'

Another lengthy silence followed. 'Is that why you've been so determined I get professional help? You're worried I might do the same thing?'

She closed her eyes. 'I guess.'

'Oh, Kate, that's not something I'd ever do. I promise you. Things have been tough, but I know they'll get better. Or at least, I hope they will. If I'd known that's why you were so worried, I'd never have been so insensitive about it. I'm so sorry.'

'You weren't to know. I'd just hate for your family to be left like ours were, confused and hurt, and wishing they'd known something was up so they could've helped.'

'God, that must've been awful.' His voice was barely a whisper.

She let out a sigh, relieved her breathing had returned to normal. 'Mind you, it's not like you've ever hidden your pain, not really. You might not want to talk to a stranger about it, but you've always been honest about your struggles with those close to you. Perhaps it's me who's being unfair. Maybe I'm projecting my experiences onto you and you're absolutely fine.'

'Hardly.'

'Well, as fine as you can be, in the circumstances.' She wiped her clammy hands on her leggings.

'Kate…? Can you open the door, please? I need to see you're okay.'

It was time to face him. She couldn't stay hidden forever.

Resigned to her fate, she shuffled onto her knees and stood up. 'I'm sorry for having a meltdown,' she said, opening the door. 'I really do love the guitar. I'm beyond touched that you got me something so special. Thank you.'

'Come here,' he said, opening his arms.

Only a fool wouldn't go to him. It was the right thing to do. Not just for her own comfort, but for his, too. They'd both been through hell. And this was their last night together. After tomorrow they would be flying solo in the world, each trying to find their path in life and recover from their trauma.

As she stepped into his embrace, breathing in his after-shave, and feeling his arms tighten around her, another wave of emotion threatened to undo her. It wasn't like the pain of losing Tristan, which had been destructive and soul-destroying. This loss was built on pure love alone. Calvin had never been anything but kind to her. Supportive. Fun. He'd made her feel capable and strong. And she'd always be grateful to him. It was an even bigger gift than the guitar.

But their embrace was interrupted by a loud bang that made them both jump.

As they sprung apart, they noticed that the window had crashed open and hit the wall, letting in a blast of cold air.

'That bloody window,' he said, shooting over to close it, only to be smacked in the face by something small and dark flying towards him. 'What the f…?' His arms flailed about, sending the creature into a terrified frenzy.

'Stop moving!' Kate cried, as she ran over. 'Stay still!' But he was in full panic mode, trying to beat the thing away.

'Get it off me!' he yelled, trying to escape the onslaught. 'What the hell is it?'

'It's a bat,' she said, trying to catch his flailing arms.

'A bat? *Shit!*' He flung himself around the room, waving his arms about, which only frightened the poor creature even more – as he was now entangled in Calvin's hair.

This development increased Calvin's panic levels, and Kate knew that if she didn't intervene soon, they might both end up falling out the window. Or worse, Calvin's heart would give out. Oh, God, his heart.

'You need to stop moving,' she said, grabbing his arms. 'Calvin, listen to me. Stand still!'

He stopped moving, even if he continued shaking like a volcano about to erupt.

'I can't help if you keep moving, okay? Now, I want you to stand very still and close your eyes. Whatever happens, focus on the sound of my voice. Can you do that?'

'I don't know.'

'Yes, you can.' She thought back to all the times he'd calmed her down and got her through a panic attack. It was her turn now. 'I promise you this will be over soon, but only if you let me help you.'

The bat continued to flap, making faint squeaking noises. 'Hurry up.'

'Just breathe, okay? Take long deep breaths and remember that the bat is a hundred times more scared than you are.'

'I doubt that.'

When she was certain he wouldn't move, she let go of his arms and moved around to his back. 'He's tiny compared to you. You're like a giant to him. And believe me, he wants out of this situation just as much as you do.' She reached up and, after a few fumbled attempts, managed to catch hold of the bat. 'That's it, nice deep breaths. I'm going to untangle him from your hair now. Keep nice and still.'

'Are you done yet?'

'Nearly.' She tried not to damage the animal as she unwound its tiny feet from Calvin's hair. 'Almost there. At least now we know why the windows keep opening. The bats must be flying into them and knocking them open. No wonder I hear so many strange noises in the night. There's probably a whole colony of them living in the roof.'

'Yeah, not helping.'

'I thought you'd be relieved. At least now you know the place isn't haunted.'

'I think I'd prefer living with ghosts than bats.'

'I didn't think you believed in ghosts,' she said, releasing the final strand of hair.

'I may change my position on that.'

'Rowan will be delighted.' Finally, she pulled the bat away. 'All done.'

'Is it out?'

'Yes, he's out. Or maybe it's a she. This could be Ursula, for all we know, disguised as a bat.' She carried the creature over to the window.

'Don't even go there,' he said, ripping off his hairband and shaking his head upside down. 'I can't deal with ghosts *and* bats.'

Kate eased the bat out of the window and watched it fly off, no doubt as traumatised as the man in her bedroom.

Closing the window, she headed into the bathroom to wash her hands. 'By the way, don't move just yet – you have bat droppings down your back.'

'Shit!' Calvin yanked at the front of his smart black shirt, sending buttons flying as he ripped it open and tore it from his body like it was on fire. Throwing the garment on the floor, he began stamping on it. 'I can't believe that bat shat on me!'

Kate stood in the bathroom doorway, gawping as she watched a semi-naked Calvin beat the shit out of his shirt. Swallowing had suddenly become a little tricky.

He swiped at his arms. 'Has it gone? Is there any on me?'

Oh, heavens.

Drying her hands on her leggings, she rushed over, fearing he was about to spontaneously combust. 'Stop panicking. There's nothing on you, I promise.'

'Are you sure?'

'Honestly, you're fine.' Faced with his bare torso, it was incredibly hard not to stare. 'There was a tiny smudge on your shirt, that's all. I was exaggerating. I'm sorry.'

'Are you sure there's nothing on me?' He turned so she could inspect his back.

She was faced with perfect golden skin, sculptured shoulder blades, a defined set of muscles sweeping over his shoulders and cascading down his back into the waistband of his jeans. Another awkward swallow followed. 'You're... perfect.' Understatement.

He turned and enveloped her in a tight hug. 'Thank God you were here,' he said, squeezing the breath out of her. 'Sorry for the meltdown.'

She was in direct contact with his bare torso and her heart began to flutter like a butterfly trapped under glass. Thank heavens she wasn't the one with the heart condition – this would have sent her into coronary failure for sure.

She thought back to that day when she'd stumbled across him naked, getting out of the shower. Here she was, a few weeks later, wrapped in those same arms, pressed against that smooth bare chest, feeling the firmness of his muscles, tasting the saltiness of his skin, and aware of every nerve ending in her body.

The hug lasted quite a while – as if they were both suffering from the comedown of an extreme adrenaline rush and reluctant to let go.

It was only as their respective heart rates subsided that things started to change. Slowly at first, a friendly hug morphing, from the platonic need for comfort, into something more primal. His fingers splayed as he explored the contours of her back, leaving a trail of heat through the thin fabric of her top. His breathing grew shallow and his lips slowly began caressing the crook of her neck, hitting a nerve that sent shock waves hurtling down to her nether regions.

Driven on by such a surge of wanting, her hands skimmed over the length of his spine, noting where each vertebra began and ended. She breathed in his scent, her tongue trailing over his collarbone…

His sharp intake of breath matched hers.

She'd licked him?

There was a pause.

He drew back and his eyes locked on hers.

The heat in his expression was nothing like she'd ever experienced before.

It didn't take a genius to work out what was coming next.

And it wasn't playing Pop-Up Pirate.

Chapter Twenty-Two

New Year's Eve

Rose Court was suspiciously quiet when Calvin jogged up the steps and opened the front door. His footsteps echoed on the stone flooring as he crossed the lobby. 'Anyone here?' he called out, depositing his suitcase by the coat stand.

'In here!' Granny Esme shouted from the dining room.

Considering how quiet the place was, he was dumfounded when he headed into the dining room and discovered everyone congregated there. The sight made him stop with a jolt. 'What's going on?' he said, looking around at a sea of expectant faces.

'Nothing's going on,' Esme said innocently, which meant that something was definitely going on. 'Your mum called to say you were on your way back, so we wanted to be here to welcome you.'

Everyone nodded silently, increasing his suspicion. Why were they so quiet?

Rowan was sitting next to Esme, clutching her hand like they were on a ship about to sink. Geraldine sat opposite, with Suki asleep at her feet. Larry, Nelson and Natalie were squashed in between, with baby Jacob lying in his portable seat.

At the adjacent table, Hanna and Alex were looking solemn, as though they expected someone to die at any moment. When he glanced over, they both gave strained smiles, which in itself was alarming.

Hanna's iPad was open on the table, Deshad's face visible on the screen.

'Did you have a good journey?' Geraldine asked, sitting bolt upright in the chair, as though she had a rod up her back. 'Have you eaten? Can I get you something?'

'I'm fine, thanks.' He scanned their faces, wondering what they were up to. They were never normally this polite. 'Okay, what's happened? Why are you all acting so weird?'

Rowan gripped Esme's hand. 'Nothing's happened. Like Esme said, we just wanted to welcome you back.'

They all nodded.

'And to see whether... perhaps, you'd made a decision about your future?' Esme said, sounding tentative.

Ah, so that's why they were all congregated in here. They were expecting an announcement. He looked around the room and realised they were collectively holding their breath. It was time to put them out of their misery.

'I have come to a decision,' he said, moving into the room. 'I'm staying in Kent permanently. I want to make a go of managing Rose Court.'

The room exploded with cheers and clapping. Everyone jumped up out of their chairs and rushed towards him, swamping him as though he'd just scored the winning goal in extra time.

'Oh, thank God!' Esme said, hugging him.

Geraldine landed a kiss on his cheek, and Rowan yelled, 'Hooray! He's staying!'

Larry slapped him on the back, and Hanna and Alex started letting off party poppers. It was carnage. Made worse when Suki started barking and Jacob started crying.

'You don't know how happy you've made us.' Esme kissed him on the cheek. 'My beautiful boy. You have no idea what this means to us.'

'We couldn't be happier.' Rowan kissed his other cheek.

With Geraldine's arms around his waist, Suki licking his hand, and Esme and Rowan hanging off his arms, he felt somewhat overwhelmed. Celebrations hadn't been this exuberant when he'd scored a last-minute equaliser in the FA Cup semi-final one year.

He was dragged over to a chair and plonked onto it. There was a loud pop when a bottle of champagne was opened, and the next thing he knew, he was seated in the middle of the huddle with a glass of fizz in his hand.

Rowan wiped away a tear. 'What made you change your mind?'

Good question.

It had been an odd week. Returning to Leeds had evoked a host of emotions he hadn't expected. As great as it had been catching up with everyone, it had also felt uncomfortable, like he no longer fitted into their world, and he hadn't expected that.

His family had been delighted to see him and relieved to find him looking better than when he'd left, but when he'd confessed his uncertainty about his future, they hadn't begged him to return to Yorkshire, as he'd predicted. Instead, they'd encouraged him to explore the opportunity in Kent, even if it wasn't long term.

'What have you got to lose?' his brother had pointed out. 'If it doesn't work out, it's no big deal. Sell the business, chalk it up to a bad experience and move on.' Wise words from his youngest sibling.

He realised everyone was waiting for his reply. 'I suppose I was unsure about taking on this place because I didn't want to let anyone down,' he admitted, deciding honesty was the best policy. 'I wasn't convinced I was in the right headspace to make a success of it. You deserve nothing less than complete commitment from whoever's running it. I had to be sure I could offer you that.'

'And can you?' Hanna's stern expression was back in place.

He nodded. 'But I can't do it alone. I'm going to need help.'

'We'll help you,' Natalie said, trying to pacify Jacob. 'You have our complete support.'

'Hear! Hear!' Rowan knocked back a swig of champagne. 'We'll all pitch in.'

Calvin smiled. 'That's kind of you, Rowan. But I don't expect the residents to help run the place. We're supposed to be looking after you, not the other way around.'

'We're not past it yet,' Esme said, giving Calvin one of her looks.

'I never for one moment thought you were,' he said, laughing.

Hanna folded her arms. 'You have money to fix things?'

'I'm getting there. Probate has been granted, so the funds will be distributed to the beneficiaries soon, and I've put my house in Leeds on the market. This means I'll be in a position to start paying regular salaries and investing in the business.' He turned to Nelson. 'You still want that full-time job?'

'Hell, yes.' Nelson gave Calvin a high five. 'Cheers, mate. Can I continue to live in?'

Calvin shrugged. 'Sure, if you want.'

Nelson glanced at Natalie, who avoided eye contact. 'I do, yeah.'

Calvin looked between them. Nelson and Natalie? But he couldn't dwell on his shock, because Hanna shoved Alex in the back, sending him stumbling forwards.

'So the thing is,' Alex said, clearing his throat. 'You're going to need an office manager. I've recently completed an online course in payroll and business management, and combined with my accountancy qualifications, I feel I have the necessary attributes to fulfil the role.' It sounded like he'd been rehearsing his speech. 'I'd like to apply for the position.' He glanced at Hanna, who nodded, confirming he'd done a good job.

Calvin smiled. 'Mate, the job's yours. You don't have to apply for it.'

Alex's eyes grew wide. 'I don't?'

'I was going to offer it to you anyway. It's a no-brainer.'

'Shit.' He sounded relieved. 'Er... I mean, thanks. That means a lot. I won't let you down.'

'I know you won't.' Calvin turned to Geraldine. 'And I'll advertise for a new chef, but can you stay on until we find a replacement?'

'Of course,' she said, smiling. 'On one condition.'

He tilted his head. 'Which is?'

'Suki stays here with you. I can't give her the exercise she needs these days, and I'm not getting any younger. It's not fair of me to keep her.'

He reeled with shock. 'I can't take your dog, Geraldine.'

'Of course you can. This is her home, and she's happier here than stuck inside my cottage. Besides, in case you hadn't noticed, she's switched allegiance. It's you she responds to now. She only listens to me if you're not around.' She placed a hand on his shoulder. 'I've made up my mind, and I want you to take her. It's not like I won't ever see her. I'd like to continue here on a voluntary part-time basis, if the new chef's okay with that.'

'I'm sure they will be. I'll make it a condition of the contract. Are you sure?'

Geraldine nodded. 'Positive. You'd be doing me a favour.'

Calvin looked down at Suki, who gazed at him expectantly, as if she was waiting for his response. 'In that case, I'd love to take her.' Suki jumped up and licked him, her tail wagging so hard she nearly knocked the champagne flute out of Geraldine's hand.

Geraldine tutted and wiped away spilt champagne. 'You're a good man, Calvin Johnson. I knew it the first moment I met you.'

'That just leaves one thing.' Larry's interruption caused all heads to turn in his direction. 'A certain young lady?'

'He's referring to Kate,' Rowan said, as if it wasn't obvious.

Calvin felt a twinge in his chest. 'I'm not sure what you mean.' But inevitably thoughts of Christmas night tumbled back into his mind. There was no way either of them could have predicted how the evening would have ended, but maybe that was just as well. If they'd had time to overanalyse the situation, they might have changed their minds. As it was, it was probably the first time since he could remember that his mind had switched off and he'd been guided by pure instinct.

What had followed was tender, passionate and so utterly gorgeous that he hadn't been able to stop thinking about it all week. It had felt like the most natural thing in the world... which was why waking up to an empty bed the following morning had been so crushing.

'We hoped she might want to stay here, with you... with us,' Esme said, softly. 'She's part of the family. We miss her.'

They all nodded.

'I miss her, too,' he admitted, his voice cracking. 'But her position here was only ever temporary. It's finished now. There's no reason for her to stay. She's starting a new job in London next week.' He glanced at Alex. 'That's right, isn't it?'

Alex nodded.

His heart sank, even though it was no more than he expected. 'It's what she wants, and I have to respect that. She's had a hard time over recent years and she deserves a break. This new job will give her financial security and help to rebuild her life. I can't ask her to give that up for me, it wouldn't be fair.'

A pause followed, with numerous furtive glances being exchanged.

'That's all well and good, but do you love her?' Larry asked, the only one brave enough to broach the question.

'Love her?' Calvin looked around at the faces staring back at him. There was no point denying it. 'I love her more than I thought it was possible to love anyone.'

Natalie took a sharp intake of breath.

Esme and Rowan gasped, and Hanna turned away, as if fighting back tears.

It was a while before anyone spoke, during which time Calvin tried to calm the ache in his chest. So much for healing: he had a second broken heart to recover from now, and the year wasn't even over.

Alex cleared his throat. 'What if the job in London isn't what she really wants?' he said, causing everyone to turn to him. 'From what she's told me, she's taking it because she thinks it's the sensible thing to do. But I know she liked working here because it meant she was her own boss. I think if money wasn't a concern, she'd want to work at that law clinic in Ashford.'

Esme frowned. 'What law clinic?'

Calvin turned to his granny. 'They hire out offices to self-employed solicitors so they can meet with clients. She liked the idea of it, but didn't feel it was something she could do when she had nowhere to live and no regular income.'

Esme looked incredulous. 'So offer her a place to live,' she said, like the answer was staring him in the face. 'Tell her she can stay here while she builds up her business. We'd all be okay with that, wouldn't we?'

Everyone nodded and made noises of agreement.

'And I don't know about you,' Rowan said, as if struck by an idea. 'But my will could do with updating. There must be others like me, people in the village who'd benefit from Kate's expertise. Maybe we could drum up a bit of business to help her get started?'

'Oh, good idea, Rowan.' Geraldine patted Suki's head. 'I need power of attorney forms completing, so add me to the list.'

'And I should get a will drawn up,' Natalie said, looking at Jacob. 'Especially now I'm a mum. I couldn't afford to do it before, but if we're going to get paid regularly from now on, it's something I definitely need doing.'

More nodding followed and murmurings of agreement.

Calvin frowned. 'What are you saying?'

'We're saying… give her a reason to stay,' Larry explained, looking at him earnestly. 'If she has a place to live and a few clients lined up, she might be tempted to try self-employment. It reduces the risk for her.'

Everyone nodded again.

'And she gets to be with you.' Larry smiled. 'That's what you want, isn't it?'

Calvin felt his throat tighten. 'More than anything.'

Larry's smile widened. 'Then make it happen, son.'

Make it happen? Larry made it sound so easy, like he had complete control over the situation and it was purely down to him. But it was Kate who had left, who hadn't been in touch. She'd made her feelings pretty clear. She wanted a fresh start. Shouldn't he respect that? 'Supposing she says no?'

'Then at least you tried,' Larry said, with a shrug. 'And you're not left wondering what might have been. Fortune favours the bold. I'm living testament to that. You think I'd have got my Francie if I hadn't shown a bit of guts?'

From the stories Larry had told him, he didn't think so.

Larry got up and walked over. 'Misery is easy, son. Happiness, you have to work at.'

Everyone turned to Calvin, waiting with bated breath to see what he'd do.

He thought back to his time in Leeds and his brother saying, 'What have you got to lose?' Maybe this applied to the Kate situation, too. What was the worst that could happen? She might turn him down and he'd be no worse off than he was now, heartbroken and missing her. But supposing she said yes…?

He turned to Alex. 'Is she still in Surrey?'

Alex nodded. 'She's staying at my mum's place. There's a big New Year's Eve party there tonight… Want me to text you the address?'

A flutter of excitement rippled through Calvin as he handed his granny the champagne flute with the words, 'Take this for me, will you? I need to be somewhere.' He stood up and ran for the door. 'Send me that address, Alex.'

Alex grinned. 'Will do, mate.'

Esme blew a kiss after him. 'That's my boy.'

Rowan started clapping. 'It's like a scene from a film,' he said, looking upwards. 'What's that, Ursula? Oh, absolutely. Love is indeed a splendid thing.'

Amongst cries of 'Good luck!' and 'Drive carefully!' Calvin raced from the room and headed outside to his car, a plan formulating in his head.

Chapter Twenty-Three

Eighty miles west of Pluckley, Kate was trying her best to put on a happy face and join in with the New Year's Eve celebrations.

She'd returned from her girlie shopping trip with her cousins, shattered from both the physical exertions of traipsing around Godalming searching for outfits, but also the emotional turmoil of pretending she was okay about starting a new job next week, when in truth, she was filled with dread. She loved her cousins, and they meant well, but she could have done without being coerced into buying clothes she couldn't afford.

Using the excuse of a headache, she'd managed to grab a couple of hours' alone time, lying on the bed and wallowing in self-pity, before reluctantly getting ready for tonight's party. Megan had loaned her a pair of strappy silver shoes to go with her new midnight blue dress, and she'd applied make-up and used her aunt's curling tongs to add waves to her hair. With the addition of silver hoop earrings and a sparkly bangle, her sorrow was hidden from view.

Pausing by the bedroom door, she glanced at the guitar that Calvin had bought her for Christmas. Getting to play every day had definitely helped tackle her anxiety levels, but every time she looked at it, she was reminded of Calvin, and that wasn't helping her to move on.

The problem was, she didn't want to move on. She knew she had to, but her mind and her heart were at odds. Maybe it would have been easier to walk away if she hadn't slept with him. As it was, the memory of Christmas night continued to torture her. If she hadn't known what it felt like to kiss him, to be pinned under him and to feel so utterly devoured by him, then maybe she could have forgotten him. But now she knew, and it wasn't helping.

As she headed downstairs, bass music thumped through the walls, making the picture frames rattle. It was still fairly early, but the house was already filled with partygoers. The dining room was laid out with masses of buffet food and a help-yourself bar.

She poured a glass of wine and eased herself through the throng of people congregated in the hallway. Judging by the size of them, she assumed they must be members of her aunty's boxing gym. There were a lot of muscled arms on display, bulging from underneath tight-fitting shirts.

The doorbell rang and Aunty Connie scuttled into the hallway to answer it. Despite being in her sixties, her aunty was a stunning woman. She'd returned from her Caribbean cruise with a glowing suntan and one of the ship's waiters – a Colombian man called Bruno, who didn't speak much English and was twenty years her junior.

'Kate, darling, go through to the lounge,' she said, shimmying past in her sequined dress, her perfume wafting into the air. 'There are some people you simply must meet.'

By this, she meant men. Kate wasn't naive enough to think otherwise. She'd overheard her aunty telling Megan this afternoon that Kate needed a 'meaningless fling' to get over Calvin. If only it was that easy.

Besides, it was the last thing Kate needed. Meaningless, or otherwise. She'd be steering clear of men for a long while yet. Maybe even forever. Because right at that moment, it felt like her shattered heart might never heal.

A song she didn't recognise blared out from the sound system her aunty had hired for the evening. Neighbours from both sides two doors down had been invited to avoid any complaints. The whole downstairs pulsated with disco lights and party streamers, and the garden had been set up for a firework display at midnight. It was quite the celebration.

Her cousins were in the lounge, standing with their respective partners. Megan looked like a screen siren in her black dress made from stretchy fabric that hugged her baby belly, her red lips and smoky eyes adding to her sultry look. She was arm in arm with her husband, Zac, ten years her junior. Like mother, like daughter, it seemed.

Beth was arm in arm with her fiancé, Matt. They'd got engaged on Christmas Day, as Kate had suspected. Matt was a firefighter, and one of the nicest men she'd ever met. She was glad her cousin had found happiness; Beth deserved nothing less.

Forcing a smile, she headed over and tried to join in with the conversation, even if her mind kept wandering back to Kent. *What are they all doing tonight?* she wondered. *Playing games? Arguing over the answers to quiz questions? Getting sloshed? All three, probably.* The thought made her smile.

And what about Calvin? What was he doing tonight? Would he be at a fancy club in Leeds, partying the night away with a load of gorgeous women? Probably.

Beth nudged her. 'Anyone would think you weren't excited about your new job. This is the answer to your problems, remember? You should be jumping for joy.'

'I am,' Kate lied, giving her cousin a fake smile.

Beth raised an eyebrow. 'You're still thinking about that legal clinic in Ashford, aren't you? I know it's appealing, but right now you need stability and a regular income.'

Megan lifted her hands in exasperation. 'God, could you be any duller? Stability is the last thing she needs. What she needs is some fun.'

Beth glared at her sister. 'Not when it comes to her career, she doesn't. She needs structure and routine.'

'She had structure and routine with Tristan, and look where that got her.' Megan touched Kate's arm. 'No offence.'

Kate forced a smile. 'None taken.'

'Now's the time to try something new. Be radical and spontaneous.' Megan winked.

'Spontaneity won't pay the rent,' Beth said, glaring. 'She needs to think about her future security.'

'I know you both mean well,' Kate interrupted, eager to prevent her cousins from coming to blows. 'And thanks for looking out for me, but I've made my decision. I've accepted that going solo isn't sensible right now, so I'm resigned to taking the job.'

Megan didn't look convinced. 'But will it make you happy?'

Kate swallowed past the tightness in her throat. 'Probably not. But I'm not sure anything would make me happy at the moment.' A tear trickled down her cheek.

Megan slid her arm around Kate's middle. 'Calvin?'

'It's silly, I know.' She wiped her eyes. 'I'm supposed to be an empowered career woman in charge of her own destiny, not a wimp crying over a boy.'

Megan looked sympathetic. 'Are you sure there isn't a future for you with him?'

Kate shook her head. 'Natalie at the care home said he's gone back to Leeds. And I'm going to be working in London, so it's never going to work. Besides, I haven't heard from him since I left Pluckley. He's made his feelings pretty clear.'

Megan wiped Kate's cheek. 'Oh, sweetie. I'm sorry.' And then her expression changed. 'Holy cow! Who's that?' she said, straining to see through the crowd. 'Talk about hot.' And then, realising what she'd said, turned to her husband. 'Not as hot as you, obviously.'

Beth tugged on Kate's dress. 'I don't like to worry you, but isn't that you-know-who?'

Kate looked over, hoping it wasn't the builder bloke from down the road that her aunty had been trying to fix her up with all week. She didn't have the energy for small talk tonight. But as the crowd parted and the man came into view, she realised it wasn't her aunty's neighbour… it was Calvin.

'Isn't that the ex-Leeds Park footballer?' Matt asked Zac. 'Calvin Johnson.'

Zac looked over. 'Bloody hell, I think it is. What's he doing here?'

'I'm guessing he's here to see Kate.' Beth gripped her cousin's hand.

'Is that him?' Megan said, sounding impressed. 'Way to go, Kate.'

But Kate was too stunned to speak. Calvin was here? At her aunty's house? In Surrey?

She realised everyone was looking at her. As if she needed reminding that the idea of her with Calvin was ludicrous. No one was more shocked than her. But why was he here?

She turned to him as he neared, her belly doing somersaults. 'Hi,' she said, unable to find anything more intelligent to say. God, she was pathetic.

'Hi,' he said, reaching her.

And then there was silence. Well, apart from the thumping music, party chatter and Megan making an appreciative whistling noise.

Her cousins and their respective partners had formed a semi-circle behind Kate and were staring open-mouthed at Calvin. Talk about excruciating.

'Hi, I'm Calvin,' he said, looking awkward as they stared at him. He was wearing a fitted black top and faded jeans, and his hair was freshly shaved underneath his curly topknot – and her heart ached at the sight of him.

Matt extended a hand. 'Good to meet you.'

Zac did the same and they all shook hands.

Kate cleared her throat. 'Sorry, I'm being rude. Calvin, this is my brother-in-law, Zac, and his wife, Megan, my cousin. And this is my other cousin, Beth, and her fiancé, Matt.'

Calvin nodded at them all. 'Good to meet you.'

Megan was making a show of giving him the once-over.

Beth nudged her sister and cleared her throat. 'Nice to meet you, Calvin. I believe you've also been working with our brother, Alex? I hope he's been behaving himself?'

'He's been great. He's a top bloke.' Calvin's eyes slid to Kate. 'In fact, I offered him a full-time job today and he accepted.'

Kate's eyes grew wide. 'Does that mean… you're staying in Kent?' Her heart rate sped up, causing a surge of blood to course through her.

Calvin nodded, his eyes never leaving hers. 'He gave me your aunty's address. I hope it's okay me showing up like this?'

The group behind her continued to stare, showing no signs of going away and giving them some privacy.

Kate managed a feeble nod, even though she still wasn't sure what him being here meant.

Calvin glanced at the faces behind her and then looked back at her. 'Any chance we could talk somewhere a bit more private?' His smile was soft and filled with warmth.

God, she'd missed his face.

Trying to regain her composure, she gestured to the patio doors. 'Outside?'

'Lead the way.' He nodded at the group, who were still staring. 'Nice meeting you.'

'Not as nice as it was meeting you,' Megan said, straining to check him out as he walked away, resulting in Beth telling her to behave.

Once outside, Kate headed down the garden path, turning occasionally to check he was still following her. Part of her wondered if she was hallucinating and he wasn't really there. But he was. In the flesh. Within touching distance. It was almost too much for her pathetic heart to bear.

The garden was lit up with strings of solar lights running down the ivy-covered walls and across the pergolas. Several people were gathered outside, despite the chill of the night, and it was hard to find a private spot, so she took him inside the summer house at the bottom of the garden, hoping it might be the one place they could be assured of privacy.

'I can't believe you're here,' she said, shutting the door and turning to him.

'Are you angry I came?' His face was cast in shadows, but she could see his uncertainty.

'Of course not. But I am a little puzzled. I haven't heard from you since… well, you know.'

He stepped towards her. 'Christmas night?'

She felt herself blush.

'I haven't heard from you either,' he said, softly.

Her eyes drifted to the floor. 'I thought it was best. You know, a clean break, and all that.'

'I wondered if you regretted it.'

'Of course not.' Her head shot up, making her earrings sway. 'How could I? It was… magical.'

He stepped closer and took her hands. 'I haven't been able to stop thinking about you. I miss you.'

'I miss you, too,' she admitted, her eyes tearing up a little.

'I hate the idea of you not being in my life.'

And just like that, the bubble burst, sending waves of sharp pain searing through her. She stepped away, sliding her hands from his, even though every instinct she had urged her to hold tight and never let go. 'The thing is, Calvin. I'm not sure that's what I want.'

His face fell. 'It's not?'

She shook her head. 'It's too painful. It was fine in the beginning, because I didn't have feelings for you, but now I do. I want to be there for you, really I do, and maybe if I was in a better place mentally, I'd be able to put aside my feelings and just be your friend. But I have to consider my own wellbeing, and the idea of seeing you and not being… you know, *with* you… is too much to bear.'

It was a long excruciating moment before he spoke. 'You think I just want to be friends?'

She blinked away tears. 'Isn't that what you're asking me?'

'No.' He stepped towards her. 'Well, yes… I do want to be friends, but I also want more than that. I want to be *with* you,' he said, taking her hands again.

She shook her head. 'You can't do. It's not logical.' She tried to remove her hands, but he wasn't letting go.

'What's logic got to do with it?'

'You and me… we're not a match.'

He looked crestfallen. 'What makes you think that?'

'You're gorgeous, and sexy, and famous. You could have any woman you want.'

'I want you.' He pulled her closer.

'Only because you're bruised and wounded from a run of bad luck.' She closed her eyes, trying to block out the sight of him, looking gorgeous, and upset, and utterly confused. 'Soon you'll be back on your feet and making a success of your life. I'm unbelievably glad you've decided to stay in Kent, as I know everyone at Rose Court will be delighted, and I wish you every happiness in the world, really I do. But let's be honest, I'm not the woman you'd choose if you were in a better place.'

'Why would you say that?'

She opened her eyes. 'Because I'm a mess. I'm homeless, skint, divorced, and I suffer with chronic anxiety. You can do so much better than me—'

He took her face in his hands and kissed her. The sudden shock sent waves of heat racing through her, and the air was sucked out of her lungs with a whoosh. Dizziness engulfed her as the room began spinning on its axis, as her senses were overloaded with the taste of him, the scent of him and the feel of his warm hands caressing her face. It was too much. The tenderness of his lips touching hers threatened to take her knees out from under her.

When he drew back, she blinked up at him. 'What was that for?'

'It was that or shouting at you.' His hands were still cupping her face. 'If you're done telling me why you're not the woman for me, can I explain why you absolutely are?'

She managed a feeble nod, her tears dripping onto his soft hands.

'I just know.'

She waited a beat. 'That's it?'

He nodded. 'That's it.' He kissed her again, another slow tender kiss that fizzled right through her. She felt punch-drunk, as if she'd attended one of her aunty's boxing sessions. Only, it was kisses, not punches, that were threatening to knock her out.

'That's hardly a compelling argument,' she said, when he pulled away. 'Even though you sell it really well.'

He smiled, his expression filled with tenderness. 'Larry told me the story of how he met his wife, and despite all the obstacles in their way, and all the reasons why it shouldn't have worked, he just knew deep down inside that she was the woman he wanted to spend the rest of his life with.' He kissed the tip of her nose, his thumbs wiping the tears from her cheeks. 'He asked me today if I loved you… and I told him I loved you more than I thought it was possible to love anyone.'

Her knees began to shake. 'You did?'

'I did.' His eyes met hers. 'When I look at you, I don't see all those things you listed. I see a woman who's funny, eccentric, compassionate and resilient. You're incredibly thoughtful and unbelievably kind. You bought me Pop-Up Pirate, for crying out loud. You make me laugh more than anyone I know, and you understand me more than anyone I know. And in case you're still thinking this is some kind of pity-love, I also really, really fancy you.'

The knee-shaking increased. 'You do?'

His eyes dipped to her mouth. 'You have no idea.' His hands slid into her hair, creating a buzz in her blood. 'Weren't you paying attention Christmas night? There's no way I'd do any of that with a friend.' He raised an eyebrow and she felt a blush hit her cheeks. 'It's taking all my willpower not to repeat some of it now.' His hands slid higher and she had a flashback of just how good last Saturday had been. 'Is there any other reason why you don't want to be with me, other than doubting how I feel about you?'

She shook her head. 'I love you. I'm crazy about you. I want to be with you.'

His eyes drifted shut. 'Thank God for that. You had me worried for a moment.'

'But it's going to be tricky, with us living so far away.' Her voice had a wobble to it.

'About that… How would you feel about living at Rose Court?'

She hadn't expected that. 'You mean, commuting to London every day?'

'No, I mean working for yourself. Remember that law clinic in Ashford you told me about? Well, if you stayed at Rose Court and shared the library with Alex as an office, then you could set up as self-employed, without having to worry about paying rent for premises. You already have three clients lined up wanting to hire your services, and Rowan's convinced you'd get a load more once word gets around the village.'

'Three clients?'

He nodded. 'Rowan, Geraldine and Natalie.'

'But won't you need the bedroom for extra staff? If you're expanding the care home, you'll need the room.' Her mind was whirring, trying to take in what he was saying.

'I've already offered Nelson a full-time job, so we're okay for the time being staffing-wise. I want to get the repairs done on the building before we employ extra staff and take in new residents, so it'll be a while before the room is needed. By which time, I'm hoping you might want to move downstairs with me. Where there are no bats,' he said, with a wry smile.

'You mean, living together? Like a couple?'

He unleashed the dimples. 'Have I mentioned I'm in love with you?'

Oh, heavens. 'And this is what you really want?'

He kissed one cheek, then the other. 'Like Larry says… when you know, you know. And I know.' His thumb trailed down her cheek. 'So, which is to be? London and a job you don't want? Or Pluckley and getting to be your own boss?'

She smiled, blinking away the tears. 'When you put it like that, it's a no-brainer.'

'So that's a yes to Pluckley?'

She nodded. 'It's a yes to you.'

He smiled with such tenderness, she wondered how she was ever going to recover. She was certainly very unlikely to get much work done with him acting as a distraction. 'I love you, Cal.'

His rested his forehead against hers. 'I love you too, Katiekins.'

And you know what?

She believed him.

Acknowledgements

Thank you so much for reading *Someone for Everyone*. I had great fun visiting Pluckley to carry out research for the book – in particular attending the Ghost Tour around the village – a hilariously spooky and fascinating experience. I didn't encounter any ghosts, sadly, but it's a beautiful area of Kent, so I enjoyed discovering the landmarks mentioned in the book and hearing all about the local legends. The landlord of The Black Horse Inn hasn't seen any ghosts either, but it's a constant puzzle as to why wine glasses keep moving about the place. Make of that what you will. I've tried to be as faithful as I can to the resident 'ghosts' of Pluckley and the layout of the area – with a couple of exceptions – the Rose Court Care Home and Ursula are both figments of my overactive imagination. What can I say? I'm a writer. I can't help but embellish.

I'd especially like to thank Jade Gani, Wills & Probate solicitor, who gave me advice about dealing with complex estates and sense-checked the legal aspects of the story. The Wishing Will Foundation is a real charity, set up by Jade, and is a valued asset to our local community.

As always, a huge thank you to my agent, Tina Betts, who is always encouraging and a huge supporter of my writing. And a big thank you to my lovely editor, Emily Bedford, who gives me such constructive and helpful feedback and makes editing a joyful part of the process. I'd also like to thank the rest of the Canelo team for supporting my books and helping to publicise them and make them the best they can be. It really is very much appreciated.

Finally, thank you to all the fabulous readers, bloggers and fellow authors for supporting my journey, sharing posts, posting reviews and generally being wonderful people. In particular, my wonderful family and drama friends, who are always the first to read my books, leave reviews and recommend them to their friends. It's incredibly humbling. Thank you!

If you'd like to follow me on social media or make contact then I'd love to hear from you:

Twitter
@tracyacorbett

Facebook
@tracyacorbettauthor

Instagram
tracyacorbett

Website
tracycorbettauthor.co.uk